*We chased after something insubstantial,
as if it might have nourished us.
We ate what could never satisfy;
we drank into oblivion.
We took what was the shadow for the real thing
and wondered why we were unhappy.*

For Lori —

EATING THE SHADOW

A Memoir of Loss and Recovery

Best wishes

C L Watson

Fenn Books and Media
Stone Ridge, New York
www.fennbooksandmedia.com

cseupel@cs.com

Also by C L Watson

The Drum and the Melody

Night Feet

LCCN 2005933973
ISBN 0-9773951-0-3

A Note on OA and Anonymity

In keeping with the twelve-step program policy of anonymity, only the
spirit and nature of Overeaters Anonymous meetings are represented,
and not the literal words or names of any participants.

Some names, places, and details in this book have been changed to
protect privacy.

Dedicated to my brother and sister-in-law

I have more flesh than another man, and therefore more frailty.

Shakespeare, Henry IV

Part One, III:3

CONTENTS

ONE: CARTER
Late February, the Present

*I*T was 9:37 p.m. My brother Carter was trying to take a bath. His wife, Lyndsey, had fallen asleep and he did not want to disturb her.

The pressure socks were a problem. His pants, the suspenders flipped easily from the shoulders, his boxers, and his shirt lay crumpled on the bathroom floor. But the tight knee socks that kept his feet from filling with fluid were difficult. Sitting on the toilet, he worked a finger under the elastic edge just under his knee. The sock started to slide down. He got the other one down, too, and rubbed his feet across his ankles so that the socks came off. The problem, of course, was not getting the socks off. The problem was getting them back on again. Maybe Lyndsey would be awake by then.

The aqua tub had a chrome bar on the side, which Carter grabbed as he stepped into the hot water. Slowly, one hand on the bar and one on the side of the tub, he lowered himself down. The hot water felt good. It had been days since he had tried to take a bath. The tub contained him like a shell around a mollusk. His huge body pressed up against the edges; his knees rose pale and smooth from the center. He draped the aqua wash cloth with the embroidered pink flowers over his knee and realized he had left the soap in the wall soap dish above the bar.

The soap dish was a conundrum. Had there been a shower in this bathroom, the soap would have been at precisely the right height. But there was only the deep aqua tub with the round, white jet portals. No shower, not even the nub of a spout for a shower. A shower would have been so much easier. Downstairs, in the other bathroom, there was a shower with a seat in it, but Carter could no longer go downstairs. Why did the people who built this house put the soap dish so high?

Already, he knew he couldn't reach it, but still he tried. His fingers climbed the wall above the chrome bar, and his other hand pressed against the bottom of the tub. His hand slipped and he fell sideways, banging his chin on the edge of the tub. He shouted, tasting blood. A great wave of water sloshed over the side. Not good, he thought, rubbing his chin and touching the place on his tongue where he had bitten it. The water was going to drip into the song room below, and Lyndsey would be pissed. Maybe she had heard him shout and she would wake up.

Lyndsey did not wake up. Carter rubbed himself with the warm washcloth, without soap. He tried to rub his back, but he could only reach the back of his neck. He caught sight of himself in the mirror, a great, hulking lump of a man, grown almost as round as he was tall, unable to reach back as if he were muscle-bound. He could take on Arnold Schwartzenager, he thought, and a rumble began in his belly and bubbled up into a raspy, breathy chuckle. He looked at the sink counter, where he had neatly aligned the shampoo, the conditioner, the back scrubber, the shaving cream, the razor, and the hand mirror, all of which were now out of reach. He laughed his raspy laugh again and pressed Lyndsey's washcloth to his mouth. His shoulders shook and tears came to his eyes. So much for cleanliness.

If he could turn over, he thought, he could probably get up. He pressed his knees to the right and grabbed the right side of the tub with his left hand. That's as far as he got. Nothing else moved. He tried pulling on the chrome bar, already knowing it wouldn't work. He braced his right hand on the side of the tub and lifted himself a few inches before falling back. More water sloshed over the side. He leaned back and rested.

The water was getting cold. He couldn't reach far enough forward to turn the hot water on again, nor could he drain the tub. He was starting to get goosebumps. A pain began in his chest, the way it might if he had been exerting himself – a weight like a stone in his breast and a shortness of breath. It was his heart. Fear broke over him in another chilly wave. "Lyndsey," he bellowed. "Lynn!"

Lyndsey appeared in the doorway, her nightgown rumpled and her red hair, the gray just beginning to streak through it, puffed up around her head. "What are you doing?" she demanded, running over to the tub.

"I need my spray," said Carter.

"Why didn't you wait for me?"

"Just get my spray."

Lyndsey got him a tiny spray bottle from his black kit on the counter. He sprayed the nitro onto the back of his tongue and handed the bottle back to her. She touched the water.

"The water is freezing. What are you doing?" she demanded again. "I told you I'd help you in the morning."

This time, Carter looked sheepish. "I didn't want to wait."

Lyndsey let the water drain out of the tub and got behind Carter. She pushed while he pulled and he rose to his feet. She wrapped a towel around him, feeling angry. She had been so tired. She had just wanted to get one good night's sleep. She was going to tell him he had to think about her needs, too, but as he sat heavily on the toilet seat, she saw that there was not water on his face, but tears.

"I'm sorry," he said.

"It's okay," she whispered.

TWO: MORE POWERFUL THAN DOGS, 1956 – 1963

I am four and a half and Carter is ten. I am standing at one end of the living room holding my baby bottle, screaming at Carter. Carter is at the other end of the living room, laughing. He is big; he is a giant to me. His round face splits with a hearty grin, and I hate him from the top of his blonde brush crew cut down to the soles of his high top sneakers. I hurl my bottle at him as hard as I can. Despite his bulk, Carter leaps behind the vestibule door with surprising agility, pulling it half shut. My precious bottle shatters into a million babyglass fragments.

"Well, that's it," says Ma from somewhere in the shadows behind me. "You're too old for a bottle anyway. That was your last one and you're not getting another."

I regret my haste and rage. I regret the vestibule door. I regret missing my brother's head.

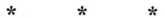

Carter is chasing me around the living room with a lit match inches from my long blonde hair. I am screaming. Somebody is laughing in the background. Somebody thinks it's funny. I figure Carter won't really light my hair on fire. Will he? But what if he does it by accident?

*   *   *

I exercise with Carter's dumbbells when he is not around. I am very small and skinny, but very strong. Carter is big and fat and very strong. My sister Caroline is already a grown up, older than Carter and in high school, reading Proust in French and peeling oranges with long, flat fingers. She is also very tall and strong. We do not fight. She holds my wrists very tightly when she is angry with me. Otherwise, she ignores me.

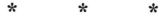

Pa has just put up a basketball hoop over the garage door. Carter is shooting hoops and I am whining about getting a turn. Another boy is there, Freddie from down the block. They shoot from the center and hit the rim; they leap and shoot from the corner and hit the backboard; they dribble the ball close and jump for a hook shot; they hit the rim. The basketball bounces into the street and some other boys from the neighborhood catch it as they stroll by. "Hey, Fatso, lower the hoop," drawls one of the boys, bouncing the ball back to Carter. The other boys laugh.

I stop whining. Abruptly, I turn and head down the block, as if I had always meant to more closely study the fir tree under which I pause. Its long branches drape over my burning face. I do not want my brother to know I heard. I do not want to augment his shame.

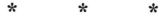

There is only one Ring Ding left, and I want it. Carter, laughing, holds it up by an edge of cellophane, higher than I can reach. I leap, again and again, screaming. Sir Toby Belch growls and barks and leaps beside me. Carter pulls the Ring Ding out of reach each time I jump. I am screaming, Toby is barking, Carter is laughing. Toby's fangs, foaming with a frenzy equal to mine, chomp into my leg. Aaurrgh, I scream, falling to the floor. Carter leans over me and I rip his face with my long, powerful fingernails. Blood wells up. Mom comes in yelling. Skin is under my nails. Nobody gets the Ring Ding.

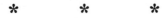

The telephone rings, and I am allowed to answer. "This is CL Watson," I say clearly. "Whom do you wish to speak to, please?"

There is silence on the other end of the line, but I can hear somebody breathing. "Poppie?" I ask. It is very late. He should have been home hours ago.

"The car broke down," he says. My father's voice is funny. Not slurred. Just … funny. The pacing is different. This happens whenever he is drunk. He always says the car broke down when he gets drunk. "Where's your mother?"

"I'll get her," I tell him. I go to my mother. "It's Pa," I tell her. "I think he's drunk."

Later, after she hangs up the phone, she is crying. I hate it when she cries. She is always crying. That's because she is weak. "I'm sure he was telling the truth," I say, trying to reassure her. "I could hear cars in the background."

She turns on me in a rage. "What do you know!" she says. "You're just a kid." She goes back to cleaning the linoleum, crying and muttering.

I turn and go to my room, holding back the hot tears. I am nothing to her.

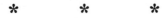

I have bitten Carter's index finger, and it is welling big gouts of blood. My mother glares at me over her glasses as she bandages Carter's finger. "A human bite is worse than a dog's bite," she admonishes sternly. Pride, fierce as any wild thing, chases through my heart: My bite, more powerful than dogs! I exult.

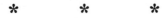

Someone has awoken Pa before ten o'clock, and he has a performance tonight. It is not one of us. Caroline is away for the summer. Carter and I are reading. We would never be so stupid.   It is the Good Humor man coming down the street. The children are shouting and calling. Ma hurries us out the back door, but still we hear his growl, black with menace. "Who the fuck is that?" he demands, shouting. Not the children, she is telling him. It's coming from outside.

Carter and I do not look at each other. I know that word, "fuck." It is a very bad word. I have never heard my parents utter such a word before. Carter has some money in his pocket. He buys me a Good Humor ice cream, Coconut Treat. Carter eats two Toasted Almonds very fast. We do not speak. It is low tide, and we wander across the street to the blunt rocks where the bulwarks end and the vacant lot trails down into the canal. The smell of the sea and salt mud lingers in the warm air.

"Thanks a lot, Carter," I say, remembering my manners. Carter says nothing.

Coconut will always remind me of Carter.

*   *   *

Pa is doing summer stock in Stratford, and he is taking me with him before everybody else. He is going to play Richard the Third, and I will watch him rehearse. I like to watch his rehearsals; sometimes I act in shows, too, though not Shakespeare. Carter and Caroline do not act. They like to play charades, though. Caroline plays the piano, too, and we all sing. That is fun, but I don't like it when Ma's trained soprano like a crystal waterfall drowns me out. I will take my notebook to the darkened theater and write poems if I get bored. I am going to go with Pa one week before Ma and Carter and Caroline arrive, so that we can be together, just the two of us. That is because we have a special relationship.

I am dancing about as Ma packs my bag for tomorrow. A lot of my stuff has name tags on it because sometimes I go to summer camp. Carter says he and Caroline never got to go to summer camp, and I am glad I get to, because I love to go away. From outside my room, where Ma can't see, Carter is throwing straight pins at me from Ma's sewing basket. I pick them up and throw them back, but one of them sticks into my foot, and I howl. Ma gets angry and chases Carter away.

Sometimes, when Pa and I are alone, he tells me that he loves me the best. He thinks he is giving me a compliment, but I hate it when he says that. It's not right. I love our special relationship, but a father should love all his children equally. He only says that when he is drunk, anyway. I am sure he loves Caroline and Carter just as much as he loves me.

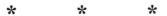

Ma's mother, Gigi, is visiting. She is very tall and has thick, white hair cut short, and she wears fashionable clothes. She doesn't look like Ma, who is small and blonde like me.

Gigi is a sharp critic. Carter disappears when she visits, and sometimes she makes Caroline cry. In the afternoon, she gets drunk and tells endless, funny stories about the wild things she did when she was a Flapper. We all thought she had quit drinking, but her little, black book called *One Day at a Time* sits in her suitcase for the whole visit. One day at a time, I am waiting for her to leave.

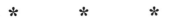

Ma and Pa have told me to call them when Carter bothers me. He cradles my body in his arms, sitting on the living room couch, one huge arm wrapped around my neck, the other under my knees, his hands clasped in front, squeezing me like a lug wrench around a nut. He pretends to kiss me, rubbing his prickly cheekstubble into my face. I am screaming for my father. Screaming for my parents to help me, but they are in the dining room reading *The New York Times*. I break free of his arms and, screaming still, rush to the kitchen, throw open the counter drawer, and grab the big, black-handled carving knife. I am going to kill him.

Behind me, a firm hand is lain on my shoulder. "CL," says my father, "that's enough."

The knife drops from my fingers like molten rock. There is a sensation in my head; it is as if I were emerging from deep water. I take a breath, more shocked than my father. What would I have done had my father not stopped me? Only I know that I was, truly, going to kill my brother. The depth of my rage frightens me. Perhaps, I think, we should try to get along better.

He is not always mean, after all. He nails cross pieces into the maple tree so that I can reach the lowest branches, from which I climb to the tippy-top, swaying in the thin leaves and surveying our Long Island neighborhood – the tarred roof tops, the vacant lots, the cattails growing near the canal, and the short street to the beach. He shows me where the best worms are, how to bait a hook, how to wait for the bite, still and silent, the hot smell of creosote and sea weed above, and the cool salt depths below. One day, he takes me to the "big beach" on the other side of town. I ride on the hard back rim of his bicycle to this foreign and exotic beach, the one where you have to pay fifty cents to get in – the teenagers' beach with a fence around it and a bathroom and a snack stand. I clutch my dollar bill and dream of frozen Milky Way bars.

*   *   *

Christmas is the best time of the year. Gifts are piled impossibly high under the tree we have all helped to decorate. Every Christmas eve, I sleep with Caroline in her big bed. We whisper into the night. I am so excited, I think I can't sleep. I am worried about Santa not showing up, but somehow sleep, like a great black horse, overtakes me.

We are not allowed to wake our parents until 7 a.m. We cannot look at the presents before they get up, but we can get our stockings. At first light, Carter creeps into our room with all three stockings and wakes us up. It is a tradition for just us three.

"Merry Christmas! Merry Christmas" Carter sings quietly, as jolly as Santa himself, holding our bulging stockings aloft. Caroline turns on her reading light, and the three of us sit on her bed and dump out our stockings. Caroline shows Carter her haul. Carter graciously allows me to poke a hole in the bottom of one of his Whitman Sampler candies before I actually taste it. I let him sample my Russell Stover chocolate-covered marshmallow Santa. Caroline sets up a game of canasta on the white bedspread, and we play cards, eating oranges and chocolate and candy canes. This is Christmas morning; it is our special time.

*   *   *

It is Sunday, and we have just returned from church. Carter is hot and thirsty when we come in, and he yanks open the ice box and gulps down a long draught of milk straight from the carton. He is always doing that. His thick neck folds back on itself, his eyes close, and his Adam's apple bobbles up and down, up and down. Ma yells at him. "Drink water when you are thirsty!" she always tells him. Drinking milk like water is expensive.

There is a hard pain in my stomach where the hunger is gnawing, but I must wait for Sunday dinner. None of my friends have Sunday dinner. I know this has something to do with my parents coming from The South, where everyone goes to church and has Sunday dinner. Carter says everything is better in The South, where he visited Uncle John on the farm last summer. People are kind and friendly in The South, he says. People are all like one big family. It is different there. Carter wishes we lived in The South.

I think people are friendly right here; I have lots of friends; I do not understand what he means. What I do understand is that every Sunday, there is a pain in my stomach until noon, when Ma serves Sunday dinner. There is fried chicken, rice and gravy, biscuits with butter and honey, iced tea with mint, corn on the cob, salad, and lima beans. I hate lima beans but I have to try just one. There is pecan pie and ice cream, or Lija May's chocolate whipped cream cake, or frozen lemon custard.

Carter always finishes what is on my plate. I am so hungry at Sunday dinner, but when I eat, not much fits. He eats the rest of my food, drinks the rest of my milk. After dinner, Carter always rubs his hands together and says, "What's for dessert?" When Ma and Pa are not looking, Carter balls up his napkin and throws it at me. We throw napkins at each other until Caroline objects.

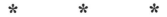

Ma and I are watching Walt Disney on TV one night. Pa is not home; he is on tour. Caroline is out with friends and Carter is at a party. We hear a scary noise at the back door. A noise like somebody playing tricks.

"Who is it?" Ma demands sharply thorough the door. "Who's there?"

We hear another sound outside, a sound like somebody saying something nasty, or like somebody blowing raspberries and calling in rude voices.

Ma throws open the door. Carter staggers, reeling below the steps. He leans over and throws up on the walk. A car full of boys drives away.

"Carter!" says Ma, guiding him inside. His clothes are covered in vomit. His eyes are open and vacant. He reels and staggers as he walks across the living room. Walt Disney plays on in black and white, unheeded. My face has gone gray.

"Mommy," I gasp. "What is wrong with him?"

Ma guides him into his room and puts a large cook pot next to his bed. She struggles to get his soiled shirt off. Carter leans over and vomits again, but nothing comes out.

"He was drinking," says Ma bitterly. "Those boys just dumped him out of the car and left him there."

All night, Carter heaves with a dry sickness.

He will drink again like this. He will drink like this every time I see him drink.

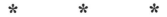

It is dark in the living room, but something has woken me up. Caroline is in there, turning off the TV. Carter has fallen asleep on the couch again. He is slouched on his side, his face turned to the wall. I can see them by the moonlight and by the light of the hall bathroom. Caroline is taking a large, framed picture of a girl from where it stuck, hidden between Carter's body and the back of the couch.

"He is in love with her," Caroline whispers to me, showing me the picture. I can see nothing but the silhouette of dark hair. "She doesn't like him. I don't know why he wastes his time."

"Why doesn't she like him?" I whisper. Caroline does not respond. "How do you know she doesn't like him?" I whisper again.

"He was crying," she whispers to me.

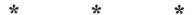

At my best friend Patty's house, a woman is visiting Patty's mother. She lives down the block. The two women sit together at the kitchen table, chatting and laughing and drinking coffee. They are dressed in shorts and midriff blouses and flip-flops. Patty tells me that this woman is her mother's best friend. I am amazed. I did not know that adults had friends.

*   *   *

I am sick with Strep Thoat. It hurts really badly, but only in my throat. Carter and Caroline say hello from outside the bedroom door. Ma runs back and forth, hovering as I lie quietly in bed with the clean, crisp sheets. She sits next to me and lays her cool, soft hand on my forehead, stroking back my hair. I fall asleep with her hands on my brow. When I wake, she brings me water and ice cream and feeds it to me with a spoon because my arms are so weak. She sits next to me and reads aloud. She massages my hands.

I love being sick.

*   *   *

We always have fun when we go to the beach. Near the ocean, Pa draws a maze in the hard sand with two sticks. It is round and curving; some passages have dead ends; some passages lead into others. We are not allowed to look at it until Pa has finished. Then we play tag in the maze, except for Ma, who likes to sit and read her book. You are not allowed to jump over the lines. We scream and laugh and other people stare at us, but we don't care. Later, Pa will build an enormous sand castle with me, decorated with seaweed and shells, with moats and turrets. Then we will ride the waves. In the shallows, I will curl up and Carter and Pa toss me back and forth like a beach ball. I will dive from their shoulders. Even though I am still small, I am getting a little too old to be tossed by them like a beach ball. But I don't say anything because they like it; it is funny and makes us close. The beach is a happy place, a place where you can laugh and feel free.

*   *   *

Carter and Freddie and a few other boys are playing football in the back yard. Carter loves football; he watches football on TV and he plays football in the back yard all the time. It's annoying because I want to go on the swings and sometimes I get hit in the head with the ball. Carter is so big and heavy, he pushes right through the other boys. They grab on to him, three of them holding his shirt and his belt, trying to drag him down, but he ploughs on to the goal, dragging them on the ground with him like big crabs that won't let go.

I assume my brother and his friends are practicing for their high school football games. It is only much later, when I am trying to understand what happened to us, that Carter tells me he did not play any organized sports when he was growing up. "I was a real nerd," he says of himself. "Caroline's boyfriend tried to get me on the football team, but nothing ever happened."

"Why didn't Carter play any sports?" I ask Caroline later on. "He loved sports. Where was Dad?"

"I don't know. Always working, always on tour," says Caroline. Caroline, who was a chronically late, brilliant over-achiever, cannot even remember Carter being in the same high school with her. "It makes me sad," she says. "I can't even remember going on the bus with him."

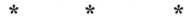

Carter and Caroline are no longer living at home. They are in college. It is very exciting when they come home. I sit in the corner of the dining room and listen as they sit at the dining room table and talk to Ma and Pa. What they say doesn't matter much. I am waiting for them to speak to me.

Carter is in something like the army in his first year at Cornell. It is called R.O.T.C., and he pronounces it "Rotsy."   Pa went to military school when he was growing up, too, before his father got fired, anyway.   I think I might like to be in Rotsy when I go to college, too.   But the next time Carter visits, he has quit Rotsy. He and my parents are arguing; Ma is crying again. Carter is going to leave school. He no longer wants to be an engineer. He doesn't know what he wants. He wants to play the guitar. He knows all the songs by Bob Dylan. He is leaving school to join the Peace Corps. I don't see Carter for two years while he builds bath houses in Iran. He has learned to speak another language.

By the time he returns, I am thirteen, and everything has changed.

THREE: THAT WHICH HIDES THE FIRMAMENT
Late February

*W*HEN I heard the phone ring at 10:27 p.m., I thought it was a B&B call. It didn't occur to me that it might be bad news about my brother. I lay in bed feeling annoyed, thinking somebody was calling our bed and breakfast in the middle of the night as if I were an all-night hotel front desk or something, instead of just a regular person who fell asleep ten minutes ago reading *The Courage to Change* with the light on and my glasses slipping down my nose and an empty Haagen Dazs container warming up on my bedside table. Furthermore, the phone was ringing in the kitchen, so I couldn't pick it up. There was no telephone in the bedroom where my husband and I were sleeping because we were sleeping in one of the guest bedrooms.

Sean and I and our two boys normally sleep in the basement. I guess you could say we live in the basement. That's where we have our telephone, beds, pajamas, clothes, uninstalled insulation, disassembled bookshelves, extra refrigerator, books, magazines, and almost everything else that we use except for our kitchen, which is upstairs on the ground floor. It is a good basement to live in, a huge basement, as big as the whole house and dry as a dusty cough. When it gets renovated, it is going to look great. I've been planning the renovation for about five years now. So far, we have a bathroom. The bathroom is done in masculine shades of gray and chrome because Sean does all of our decorating as well as all of our renovating. I figure the entire job might be finished in time for my funeral.

We did live in the house proper for one year after we escaped from New York City to this dreamhouse in the woods. We all had bedrooms with real closets. We had a kitchen and a dining room and a living room and I even had a writing office in which to eat my ice cream privately as I mused over the mysteries of life. Then reality set in, taking the form of a drained bank account. My writing assignments hit a slump and Sean's architectural woodworking business in the city was falling apart because he couldn't stand leaving us all the time to take care of business. That was when we came up with the idea of opening a B&B.

This very room in which I lay listening to the shrill ringing from the kitchen used to be our bedroom, at which time it did have a telephone. Some people might have found it difficult to give up such a bedroom to commerce, but not I. I loved revisiting its uncluttered, clean lines, the fresh linens subtle with roses and the downy comforter edged in sateen. If it were still our room, we would not have subtle roses on the sheets. We would, no doubt, have striped sheets. Probably *gray* striped sheets, with a gray comforter – since, I believe, comforters don't usually come in chrome. And it would be chaotic, too, because tidying our part of the house is very low priority in my pantheon of chores. We would have books and magazines and newspapers piled on the nightstands and the floor, clothes boiling out of the bureau drawers, pictures propped on the vanity. The room would vanish. I would no longer be able to see its beauty; it would be just another place to sleep.

But this night I was a guest in my own room. Isn't that our true state on earth, anyway? I am most myself when I am a guest. I am most present when I am a guest. I appreciate everything more when I smell it and touch it and taste it with a visitor's temporal senses.

Besides, I am mercenary and I love making money. I used to scorn money, but that's when I was young and naïve and a poet. After about fifteen years of being a young, naïve poet who scorned money, I suddenly realized that I had become an old, naïve, penniless poet. And this was the cruel thing: *You can't have a home and a family without money.* Well, I guess you could have a family, but you couldn't have a home, and what kind of life is that for a kid? That was when this poet learned how to write commercial copy. I thought of the artistic transition as a biological imperative.

Sean was already asleep and there is very little in this life that shakes him from that state once he is in it. His thin, handsome face was obscured on top by the pillow scrunched over his eyes and on the bottom by his new beard, which was growing too bushy and jutted up like a bramble. The only tender part of his body exposed to the icy air trickling into the room from the cracked-open window was his nose, which quivered with aquiline sensitivity in the fresh oxygen. Sean heats up like an engine at night, which is why he is exasperatingly thin even though he eats more sweets than I do.

My own nose, the circulation impeded by the fallen glasses, had grown chilly. The house was certainly much too cold to go running into the kitchen to answer the telephone. Instead, I took off my glasses, put the dirty spoons into the empty ice cream carton, turned out the light, and wiggled closer to Sean.

The answering machine had finally picked up the call. Idly, I listened to my own over-loud message welcoming callers and detailing the availability of rooms, and then I heard the voice of the caller, sotto, which reached me only in desultory phrases.

Suddenly, it dawned on me that something was wrong. This dawned on me only after I realized that the voice of the caller belonged not to some stranger inquiring about room availability, but rather to my elder sister, Caroline.

Caroline never calls after ten p.m. She doesn't even call after nine p.m. Caroline conks out at night even earlier than I do. This is not because she is substantially older than I, nor because she works even harder than I, but because she sleeps in a bright apartment with her airy windows so buff, the sun strikes her in the face as soon as it cracks the heavens. We Watsons liked our morning light strong; it works almost as well as a bolus of Prozac.

A call from Caroline at 10:27 p.m. did not bode well. Now I wanted to hear the message even less. There was too much bad news in our family; I didn't want to know it. In the mellow, moonlit dark, I scrunched down deeper into the warm pocket of covers, sliding my feet down Sean's even warmer legs. He shifted slightly in his sleep, bending his body into the curve of mine, sliding an arm over my belly. He hates it when I warm my ever-cold feet on his body and normally he won't let me do it, but he was vulnerable in sleep.

Caroline's voice rose and fell from the answering machine in the kitchen. I couldn't hear the actual words, but I could hear enough of the sound and the tone to know it was she. It was something bad that she wanted to discuss, but it was not an emergency. If it were an emergency, she wouldn't leave a message. She would hang up and call back right away. She would keep calling until I answered.

After a long, long time, I heard a shrill *beep*. She had left her message of any length, and she had gone off to sleep. The phone did not ring again. That meant nobody was dead or dying.

Tomorrow, I thought.

I tugged on the covers, and a puff of warm darkness wafted across my face like a mother's sigh. The night was again a living stillness, composed of calm: the slow rise and fall of Sean's chest on my back, the folds of the warm covers holding my body, the dim light illuminating the edge of the window sill. Outside, the wind *woo-wooed* as it combed the fir trees.

The bedroom door squeaked, and there were footsteps. It was our younger son, Byron, pitter-pattering into our room. No matter where Sean and I sleep, Byron can find us unerringly. He wades through broken, restless nights, and sometimes he sleepwalks with awful nightmares. I worry terribly about my little boy. There is something wrong; something deep in Byron that sees too much: some assurance missing, some vision that makes him depressed. It had started when he was just a toddler. He has inherited the family disease for sure, whether because of our mistakes or our genetics, I do not know.

However, as Byron came into the room, I realized that he was not sleepwalking. If he were, he would not have walked directly into our bedroom. Instead, I'd have heard the little steps in the living room, or maybe upstairs, running first this way and then that. Quick, then hesitant. Searching. Fleeing. Byron sleepwalking, his delicate, wiry body awake, his mind asleep, lost in his own home, eyes wide open seeing *The Horror*. No good that Mama is standing right in front of him, even holding him while he desperately looks for safety. In nightmare, he sees nothing out here where I am, hanging onto good old reality for him. He hears nothing. Only what is behind the scenes.

No nightmares tonight, though; he was just scouting for a cuddle. I lifted my head and raised the edge of the downy envelope. Byron slid in without speaking, curled up into the belly part of me. Sean's fingers settled over him, like a feather briefly disturbed. I cupped Byron's body, my arm resting on his hipbone and shoulder, so that it would not be too heavy, and the universe closed its giant eye.

We slept.

FOUR: THE MESSAGE
Late February

I forgot the message was there until after I took the boys to school. Early morning was a big rush in our house because everybody slept as late as he or she possibly could, except Sean, who had to get up before five when he was working on a union job, and he made up for it when he got laid off with his heroic ability to sleep though every kind of chaos known to man.

My older son, Harry, aged ten, jumped up with alacrity, threw open the doors, turned on all the lights, dressed, ate and brushed his teeth within seconds, and then settled down on the computer to the serious business of *Alien vs. Predator*. Byron, Harry's younger by exactly two years and three hours, was still groping his way to the bathroom. Between trying to find socks, wake Byron, make lunches, brush my own teeth, feed the animals, warm up the car, and pry Harry off the computer, there was precious little time to think about late night messages.

But to be perfectly honest, the morning rush was not the only reason I forgot the message was there. As the Great One said, our life is but a sleep and a forgetting, and I seem to specialize in both. If I can't sleep through the pain, I seem to have a knack for forgetting it even exists. So it was not until I returned from taking the boys to school (missing the school bus every day gave us a full half-hour's extra sleep) that I caught sight of the blinking number, the red "1" inside the black answering machine, blink-blink-blinking to be heard.

The answering machine hung on the wall of the kitchen in plain view so I wouldn't forget about it. Hateful thing! It used to be that you could live in present time, in real time. If they didn't get you right then, man, you were *gone*! Now we must live in double time, triple time. Deal with the past, the present, and the future, and don't forget to go to the bank. I get even more resentful when I call somebody else who *doesn't* have an answering machine. How dare you miss my call! Don't you realize that I might have something *important* to tell you? Can't I dump my problem into your lap right now and wait for *you* to deal with it?

My heart sank as I wondered what the message was. Sean was already gone for the day; otherwise I'd get him to listen to it for me. But I couldn't even call him. He was off on a union job somewhere or other, and I couldn't get in touch with him unless it was a major immediate near-death situation or worse.

A quick mental inventory covered whom I might call, depending on how horrible the news was. My old friend Hannah at her New York City office if it were about my one and only niece, Emma, because Hannah was there twelve years ago when my niece was seventeen and first developed schizophrenia. My friends Annie and Doreen if it were about my mother: Annie because we grew up together and she was like another sister, and Doreen because she was my good buddy and close neighbor.

If Caroline's cancer had come back, I'd call Annie, but if Caroline was just depressed about something, I would probably call Doreen because she always had wonderful advice that made me feel better, or I might call my friend Denise, because she was good to complain to and commiserate with.

Thus prepared, I washed a couple of dishes.

Since I hated doing housework, there was no illusion that I was doing anything except procrastinating. Finally, after scrubbing the sink with *Comet*, washing the stove tines on the range top, and finishing my most-important-meal-of-the day (two king-sized mugs of coffee with hot skim milk and sugar-substitute), I listened to Caroline's message. She spoke for three minutes and forty-five seconds by the digital clock on the stove.

"Hi, CL," her message began. She sounded ordinary but not cheerful, which meant she was anxious. But she wasn't crying, which meant she wasn't depressed. So far, so good.

Certain promises, Caroline recalled for me, had been made, certain pledges to visit Boston to see my brother, Carter, and herself. When Carter was not well enough to come to my house with Caroline and Mom and Emma for Christmas, I had said then that I was going to visit him in January or February.

It was true, I thought guiltily. February was almost over, and I had not even begun to plan a visit. Everything had been so hectic. It was so exhausting to drive six hours to Boston with the boys going crazy in the back. It was so hard to get away. I had to work on my book. I had to revise an article that had been dragging on for months. I had to take the Bed and Breakfast reservations, update the website, and plan around guest schedules. I had to do the grocery shopping, make the meals, cook for the B&B. I had to prepare my older boy Harry for his fourth-grade standardized tests. I had to drive down to New York City every Monday night to teach at NYU. I had to convince the PTA to sponsor a science fair. I had to create a strategy so that I didn't have to chair the PTA science fair myself. I had to attend the school board's meeting about the new zero-tolerance district-wide discipline policy that everybody was talking about. And speaking of discipline, I had to take our 45-pound puppy, Rue, to dog-obedience classes with Byron to teach Byron how to control him without any torture involved.

Not to mention the fact that it could be stressful to visit Carter.

"I spoke to Mom about Carter," Caroline's voice went on. She had finally gotten to the nub of the issue, the real reason she was anxious and calling me at 10:27 at night to leave me a long message. "You know," she said, "Mom just got home. She was visiting Carter this week. So she was telling me ... Evidently Carter is doing pretty badly. He's having trouble walking. Lyndsey has to help him just get around the house, now. She has to help him get dressed. Mom said he has to stop and sit down after he goes up the steps to the living room to catch his breath. She said he's over four hundred pounds now. *Lyndsey has to help him take a bath.* So if you want to see him, I think you better go soon."

If you want to see him, you'd better go soon.

Have you ever had that sensation when your skin seems to separate from the rest of your body? Your skin goes cold and prickly and it feels like it's kind of lifting off. It lifts and shivers and shakes, leaving the body numb. I could hear my own heart beating. Silence waffled against my eardrums, like blowing on a microphone. Something grazed past me: the hot bullet of my brother's death. I could feel it.

"He's over four hundred pounds now," Caroline repeated as her message continued. "I guess that diet he was trying didn't work. Call me."

Four hundred pounds. The number lay before me as if an absolute, like a thin and irrevocable line over which Carter had passed, as cold and deadly as a black garrote. I could not imagine a person weighing over four hundred pounds, and it shocked me as much as it evidently had shocked Caroline.

I was mooing around in the kitchen, not calling Caroline back, when my mother called me.

"I just got back from Carter's," she said.

"Uh-huh." I didn't mention Caroline's call. I wanted to hear Mom's version.

"Well, Carter's not doing too well."

"Yeah?" I urged.

"Well, he's kind of housebound now. He can't walk from the car to the house."

"He can't *what?*"

It was four, flat steps from Carter's car to his house.

Mom's voice was matter-of-fact. "Well, he can't walk more than a few paces without gasping for breath. You know, I think he might be over four hundred pounds now. He's having trouble dressing himself."

She *knew* he was over four hundred pounds. She was the one who told Caroline.

There was a silence on the telephone.

"Ma," I asked her, "how are you doing? Are you okay?"

"Oh, I'm doing fine," she replied with her usual brisk energy. "I'm not too tired." She had just driven home over two hundred eighty miles in three and a half hours. She speeds and refuses to wear a seat belt. Mom has more energy than any of her children. Since Mom and I look a lot alike, I'm banking on having lots of energy when I get old.

"No, I mean how are you doing with all of this with Carter ..." But

I couldn't bring myself to use the D-word. I couldn't say, "about to die." So instead I said, "…with Carter doing so badly."

Now the quaver came into her voice, but she continued stoutly. "Well, there's nothing we can do. We just have to accept that. We just have to take it one day at a time. There is nothing we can do. I know he could die any day. Any day, he could die. But it's just one day at a time. We have to be grateful for every day."

Mom was falling back on her Al-Anon training. In Al-Anon, you recover from a terminal desire to fix things – especially the alcoholic in your life. Above all, Al-Anon teaches that you cannot save anybody who doesn't want to be saved.

I understood all this, but I couldn't help wonder: Was there nothing we could do? *Nothing* we could do? The thought rankled. How can you just let somebody you love die of obesity, something that might have been prevented?

"You know," said Mom, "he's lived the way he wanted to live. He didn't die in Vietnam."

Carter didn't go to Vietnam. He was not even in the service. But I knew what she was thinking. She was trying to justify it, trying to make sense of this useless waste of life. Searching for a firm place on which to alight and steady, a place which offered some measure of equanimity.

"He didn't go to Vietnam and he didn't die there," Mom said, "or get lost forever down there like my cousin Byron, and nobody ever found his body. That could have happened to him."

Seen in this way, instead of being pissed off that Carter was dying of self-inflicted obesity, we could feel glad and grateful that he'd had so many extra years of life. I tried to feel happy that a brick hadn't fallen on his head.

"I took a lot of pictures," said Mom. "It was a good trip." Mom was a wonderful photographer. She was also a poet and a retired English teacher and a ceramist and reader and an art-appreciater and a truly amazing singer, and, in my opinion, a frustrated artist. She was probably a better actor than my father was, but she got pregnant with Caroline and that was the end of her career. It wasn't until I was grown up that she discovered her *metier*: photography. She was never without a camera.

The phone beeped. "Can you hold on, Ma? I have a call coming in."

"I'll just let you go," she said hastily. "I know you're busy."

"I'm not that busy, Ma."

The phone beeped again. I had to pick it up because it might be a B&B call.

"That's okay, I don't want to keep you," she said, ready to erase herself off the page if it might help her children.

"I'll call you back," I sighed.

"Okay. Tomorrow's okay. Love you."

I clicked over. It wasn't a B&B call, it was Doreen. Perfect timing. I told her everything.

"The only thing is," I said, "I think it might be too late to help Carter. This has happened so many times before. He has a huge health crisis, and I want to do something about it, you know, I want to help him somehow, but then I think that it's too late. And then he doesn't die; he gets better again! And the next time he has a big crisis, I'm really sorry that I didn't do something about his weight and his overeating when I was motivated after the last crisis and I think: Well, now it's *really* too late."

The incredible thing about Doreen is that she could understand exactly what I was talking about.

"You have to go ahead and try to help him this time," she said. "You can't think about if it's too late or not. Because you really have no way of knowing what's around the next corner. You can't know what will happen. Just do it. A miracle could happen! We never know what we are put here for."

She didn't use the G-word with me, but I knew what she meant. I hate all that God stuff Doreen believes in. It seems absurd to me to imagine that some benevolent presence is watching over us, giving us purpose. I hate it because I wish it were true.

"Maybe if he loses just a little weight," she went on, "maybe that could make a difference in the quality of his life. Maybe if he only lives another five years, he could still enjoy things in a way that he couldn't have otherwise. You just can't know what's in store for him."

"Another five years?" I said, dismayed. "I think he might die to-night."

Carter had explicitly said to Caroline and me that he chooses to continue to eat. He'd had it with diets. He did not feel that life was worth living if he couldn't enjoy food, and if it killed him, so be it. But I knew darn well there was a lot that Carter enjoyed besides food. He loved to fish in mountain streams; he loved to camp and backpack; he loved to play with his nephews and nieces; he loved to ski; he loved to sing; he loved to dance; he loved to celebrate life. And he loved his wife.

I couldn't help but believe that Carter was killing himself with addiction, not food. I thought something was terribly wrong, something we couldn't see. I thought he was committing suicide, but slowly, and that underneath, he was crying out for help. I didn't believe that Carter really wanted to be dead. I didn't believe he would rather die than give up eating whatever he wanted. I believed it was the addiction that wanted him dead: the compulsion itself. I pictured the addiction, that green, slimy layer of self-hatred wrapped around a small, naked child like a rotting cabbage. I believed that buried under all the anger and self-righteousness, buried under the need to control and fear and the compulsive eating and the diet-cheating, there still lurked a loving, over-weight little boy who was crying out for help – confused, frightened, and alone. I'd been there myself. How could I not answer?

"Go ahead and do it," said Doreen. "You never know."

FIVE: PERCHANCE TO DREAM, 1965

*M*Y parents are arguing in the game room. Pop is drunk again. To sleep, to sleep forever would be good. The trees, my old friends, offer me no solace this night; the dark summer air, faint with the tang of the sea, only haunts me. My parents catch sight of me and start yelling. Why don't I help? Why don't I clean up my room? Wasn't I already told to clean up my room? In the bathroom, I search again for the sleeping pills. There is only cold medicine, but these pills make you sleepy, too. They would, if you took a whole bottle or more, make you sleep forever. I am so tired; I would like to go to sleep and never wake.

There is nothing left for me now. For the past year, living in Toronto where Pop was working on a TV show, I dreamed only of returning home to my friends. It was strange and difficult in Toronto, where they made fun of my blue ice skates and my Yankee clothes and the way I pronounced "water." I had no friends in Toronto.

But when we return to Long Island, it seems I still have no friends. Everything and everyone has changed. My girlfriends have grown strange; the boys they like are older, rough and frightening. Worst of all, my best friend has become best friends with another girl. She doesn't seem to even realize it will hurt. "Me and Ellen are best friends now," grins my former best friend Patti.

I no longer fit in here. I can't even imagine what might make things better. There is no place in the whole world for me now. I am thirteen, and I am alone.

Each visit to the bathroom, I swallow more pills. Pills are easy to swallow; I've always taken three or four aspirin at a time for my migraines. I take all the cold tablets in one bottle. Then I start on the next bottle. I tuck a poem into the pocket of my pajamas. It is my suicide note. I will go to sleep, I think. I will go to sleep and never wake up. They will find the note.

Instead, I wake up in the dark, terrified. My heart jitters a million times a second. I leap out of bed and press my hands to my chest, feel the pulse in my neck. My heart is banging unnaturally, impossibly fast, banging like a runaway railroad train. How could a heart even go so fast? My body is poisoned, and I am sure I am about to have a heart attack. In a sweat, I run to the bathroom and vomit. I am dying, I think. I am dying, and I do not want to die *at all*. I run to my parents' bedroom, calling out as I run through the dark house: *Maaaaaammieeee*. The terror revs my voice into a shriek.

In bed, my parents throw the covers back and turn on the lights, their faces blanched in the sudden brilliance.

"Oh, I'm so stupid," I moan. How can I tell them?

"What's the matter?" they both urge.

I blurt it out, too frightened to hold back. "I tried to kill myself."

"What?" my father gasps. His face is a mask of horror.

I tell them about the pills. I am panting, and I don't want to die. "Am I going to die?" I ask them breathlessly. "No," Mom says in a cold, stern voice, as if challenging Death to threaten her authority, "you're not going to die."

Immediately, I feel better. The wild crashing of my heart subsides a little. Mom will save me. Mom knows what to do. My parents call the hospital and they are told to bring me in. I lie down on the back seat of our old Chevy, hanging over a mixing bowl Mom has placed on the floor. A policeman stops my father for speeding and running red lights on the long, black, deserted road. He takes one look at me throwing up in the back seat and gives us an escort. The siren wails all the way to the emergency room.

Behind a curtain in a half-darkened room, I lie in a hospital bed alone, dazed and nauseated. A nurse arrives every half hour to administer a large glass of water. It is too late to pump my stomach. Each time I drink, I throw up again. "You keep that water down," the nurse threatens, "or we'll have to put the IV back into your arm again." I long for the

IV. The nurse does not understand that I am not afraid of needles. After I vomit once again, she takes the pan from me and says, "Well, are you proud of what you've done?"

"No," I reply wearily, turning away with shame. I had always thought nurses were healers and helpers. But this woman is just like all the rest.

The next day, many young doctors crowd my hospital room curiously, asking me questions. They are polite, and ask permission before they pick up something I've been writing in my notebook. I like having so many young men pay attention to me, even though it's a little embarassing. I think I must be an important patient. I've been told that I am lucky they put me into the children's ward, even though I'm already thirteen. They've done this so I will not carry a permanent record of my suicide attempt.

Later, a nice doctor who interviews me privately asks me why I did not tell my parents I felt depressed.

This is a new concept. It has never occurred to me to speak to an adult about how I feel.

"Do you want to go to a psychiatrist?" my father says to me in the car going home. "The doctors said you should go to a psychiatrist."

"No," I say. Nobody I know goes to a psychiatrist. Nobody my parents know goes to a psychiatrist, either.

"Why did you do that?" my father asks.

"I don't know. I heard about a girl who tried to kill herself with aspirin."

They say nothing. We never mention it again. Nobody knows my permanent record. Nobody finds the note.

SIX: THE THEORY OF DOG MIND
March

A light snow had started and the air looked blue. I sat alone at the kitchen window, drinking coffee, looking out. What might save Carter?

I had been mulling it over for a week. What could I do? How did you make a seriously obese person change? What if losing weight wouldn't help Carter now, anyway?

I had not spoken to Carter yet. The thought of calling him filled me with anxiety. What would I say? Could I say anything that would make a difference? Finally, I called Carter's wife Lyndsey, The Source.

"I'm sure it would help him if he started eating right," said Lyndsey. She was at work, so we could talk freely. She was a singer and she worked part-time in an office so she could run her River of Song program at home.

"He uses the insulin to enable his eating stuff," she said. "He'll take a shot of insulin so he can eat whatever he wants to."

"Won't that make him worse?"

"Well, yeah," said Lyndsey. "You're not supposed to use insulin like that."

I thought of the time when I was visiting Carter and he got some diet Coke out to drink with our dinner. "Carter," I had said to him, aghast, "that soda has caffeine in it!" Carter had a heart condition, and he was not supposed to have caffeine.

He was blasé. "Oh, a little bit won't hurt me," he had said. I had mentally shrugged. What did I know? That night, after Lyndsey had come home and I had gone to bed, I woke to the sound of Carter moving about, talking to Lyndsey. "I had that soda with caffeine," I heard him confess to her. He sounded like a chastened child. "How could you do that!" said Lyndsey. Later, in the wee hours of the morning, she drove him to the hospital. Oh, *a little bit wouldn't hurt him!* How could he be so dishonest with himself? Carter, the hospital prisoner, doing time for the crime of being self-deceived. He was out again the next day. The revolving doors of hospital justice.

"I just think I have to do something, Lyndsey. I don't think I can live with myself if he dies and I never really tried to do anything. I want to do an intervention."

"Well, *you* know about intervention," said Lyndsey nervously. "I don't really know anything about that."

I first heard about interventions when my mother did one with my father. She wanted all of us to sit in a room and confront my father about what he had done to us to try and get him to stop drinking. I felt guilty about not participating, but at the time, I needed to "help" my parents like I needed a hole in the head. That's why I understood Lyndsey. Sometimes, it's all you can do to maintain your own stability.

I did know interventions don't always work. Can you *force* an addict to face the truth? Not really. Some choose to live; some choose to go on dying. For some addicts, the bottom they hit is stone cold dead. And even after the grave, they'd probably keep going if they could. "Man," they'd say, "Death! That was really close!"

Mom ended up doing her intervention with my father by herself. I guess all of her years in Al-Anon paid off, because it worked. My father went to AA, got sober, and became a man you might really want to know. I thought of him then as the person he was meant to be. As if before, he'd been so twisted you could only catch glimpses of any good stuff refracted off a momentary surface, and now all the little fragments of good he'd ever been had melded together into one solid human being.

Wasn't that worth it?

"Lyndsey," I said, "I don't know if this is going to work, but I gotta do it. I've just got to try."

Lyndsey didn't get it. How could anyone make Carter do anything he didn't want to do? "Why an intervention?"

I hated to tell her the truth. Maybe she'd leave him, and then what?

"If I'm going to be really honest with you, Lyndsey, I have to say that I believe that Carter is an addict, exactly the same as an alcoholic or a drug abuser, and that he is crying out for help. He can't stop himself and he needs somebody to give him a big slap in the face, you know, a real kick in the butt. Somebody has to make him face the truth. He is such a jerk when he gets angry, he gets everyone intimidated; he bamboozles everybody. He intimidates me, too. He gets so angry and is so forceful that everybody gives in to him. He needs somebody who won't give in."

"I can't do it." Lyndsey's voice was filled with regret.

"It's okay. I'll do it," said big macho me, the Charles Dickens of chickens.

Lyndsey gave me the names of Carter's doctors, and I started calling. There was the cardiologist, the general practitioner, the kidney specialist, the nurse-practitioner/nutritionist, the other really nice but far away cardiologist he still saw once in a while, the diabetes guy, and the pulmonary specialist. No one, of course, was available to speak with me. I left messages for them to call me back.

By now I had missed my exercise class and I was into my time-slot for correcting papers and preparing for my business-writing class. Soon I would have to leave for the city, and I felt all disorganized. I couldn't concentrate. I wandered to the computer and started searching the Internet for resources related to obesity. There was nothing on "compulsive over-eating." It didn't exist as a category. For "obesity," all I could find were diets. I emailed a letter to Richard Simmons, the sprightly weight-loss guru, who promised to answer personally in a couple of months. I imagined Richard Simmons in a sweaty jumpsuit jogging in front of my brother, waving his arms above his head, urging Carter to love himself. Carter growls and punches Richard in the stomach. Richard e-mails me with tears in his eyes: *"There's nothing I can do!"*

I sat with tears in my eyes, realizing that I was procrastinating about preparing for my class. And that's because I hated this particular class. Usually, I love my class, but in this particular class, I had a situation – a situation that turned out to teach me something important in my quest to help Carter.

*   *   *

I didn't know how to deal with it, and even more important, I didn't *want* to deal with it. The situation was a contingent of four students – one third of my international graduate business writing seminar at NYU. What had drawn them together was not a shared language of homeland, but rather the shared language of arrogance. They were led by a young Brazilian woman who was absolutely stunning, the kind of woman Annie and I would have hated in high school for being not only beautiful and smart, but also *tall*; the kind of woman my brother would have resented for setting her sights on somebody "better" than he. She spoke four languages and she was always talking. These students are *mucho pissedo* that they have to take my class, which I saw as a lynchpin to success and they saw as degrading remediation.

"I didn't know on the GMAT," said their leader in sonorously accented English. The others agreed. "I just rested when you had to write the essay. I didn't even try to write it! The test proctor said it was not important."

I couldn't imagine why anyone would think that an entire section of the graduate school exam doesn't count, but I didn't doubt her word.

"How about this," I said, raising my voice to blanket their querulous, self-righteous complaints. The other two-thirds of my students were slumped around the seminar table staring into space. "I'll ask if you can test out of this course. I have to speak to the head of my department. I'll give you a test and if you do okay, you don't have to take the course."

Why not, I thought. I'd be happy to see them go. They already failed to believe me when I told them that they would learn a lot even if they *could* write. I had too much to do just to help Carter; I didn't need extra grief from this crew.

The rebellious ones expressed effusive gratitude. They'd already complained to every official at school and nobody else would even give them the time of day.

The only trouble was, when I got to school that night, the head of my department said no. "That bunch," Sid said. "They've talked to everybody in the whole school. What do they expect? They flunk the GMAT, they've gotta take the course. They've already taken a test! They failed."

Easy for him to get tough. He didn't have to deal with them. But I was not surprised. Sid was a pugnacious guy who usually said exactly what was on his mind. "Fuck them," he said. "Why do they get special dispensation?"

I really liked Sid. He didn't put on airs. He didn't pull punches. You gave him a fight, and he'd be right there. He didn't back off. He was not intimidated. When I got to class, I was going to blame the whole mess on him.

But once I got there, I found that the Brazilian Queen's quartet had stopped complaining. They'd bowed to the inevitable. Their cries had been heeded. They accepted the verdict that they must abide with grace. They were no longer into fighting.

Now they were into fooling around.

Like children, they kept an eye on me as they passed something to each other under the table. Every few seconds, my profundities on the structure of the paragraph were punctuated by a whisper, a murmur, a giggle, a glance at me. It was incredibly irritating. What were they doing, passing notes? I could recall doing a little note-passing myself – in seventh grade. Even the other students were irritated, shifting restlessly in their seats and glancing at the offenders.

The pressure was building in me. My ears were getting hot. I was not sure what I was going to do. One of the four, a Russian student, revealed what they'd been passing: a rolled down paper bag. He popped something from the bag into his mouth.

I stopped the lesson and stared pointedly at them. All eyes on me. I smiled what I hoped was wickedly. "Well," I said, with a broad gesture toward the other side of the seminar table, "now you have to share your candy with the rest of the class."

The rest of the class laughed. I waited until the Russian sheepishly offered the candy to the rest of the students, who were, in fact, just as multilingual and international as the miscreants. Politely, the other students refused. I was dumbfounded when, not ten minutes later, this same student was carrying on a conversation with another one of the Fabulous Four. I stopped the class again. "Excuse me, Vladimir," I said, having glanced at my attendance sheet to find his name. *Vladimir. Stiff hair,* my notes said. "Will you please stop talking?"

Vladimir apologized with an unctuous smile. *Oh, yes, oh dear,* his smile seemed to say. *You were lecturing weren't you? Ha, ha, so silly of me, I didn't notice!*

I gave him my own version of the overly sweet smile. "Why don't we chat a little after class?"

When his cohorts were waiting for him in the hallway, Vladimir was a lot more tense. I paused, savoring my moment of power. If I failed him in the class, he couldn't get his MBA and make tons and tons of money in International Finance. Why couldn't I be this stern with Carter when he behaved like a child?

"I'm sorry," he said immediately. "It won't happen again."

I invited his friends in from the hallway. Now they were all tense.

"Look," I said to them. "If you don't want to take my class, don't come." I had been told my angry face is stone, and my eyes are stone, but to me, it felt hot and charged, like electricity crackling in and out of my dermal pores, like Bride of Frankenstein. Self-righteous anger is great. I felt fluffy and huffy, and it was comforting to know I looked scary.

"No, no," they all protested at once. "It's great! Your course is great. Sorry, sorry." And so on. They had already completed two weeks; they certainly didn't want to start all over again.

"If you want to listen, there's plenty you can learn. But I can't teach with you distracting everybody."

Again, apologies. Promises.

After that, these guys were my best friends. They fawned over me. They loved me. They handed in fabulous papers. They participated in class. They were teacher's pets.

So here was the lesson: You gotta put up your dukes. It was just like Sean always said. You gotta show 'em they can't push you around. Sean grew up dirt-poor on the tough side of the city, always brawling to save his skin. He couldn't understand the new attitude of zero-tolerance on fighting. "Some of the guys I fought with became my best friends!" he would say. "You don't have to win. You just have to show they can't push you around."

Standing in my classroom, the Theory of Dog Mind crystallized for me. Our puppy, Rue, now five months old and a little heavier than my son Byron, was perpetually seeking to establish dominance. Anything living and smaller, Rue attempted to stand on top of. Sometimes he even tried to dominate dead things, too, like tin cans and door mats. Humans (men in particular) are similar to dogs in this way. They just gotta know who's top dog. For example, at first, when Rue got big, Byron hated him. He was afraid. But then they started to tussle. First Rue was on top, then Byron was on top. Byron wrestled him to the ground, Rue rolled over on him, Byron rolled over on Rue, Rue scratched him, Byron bled and cried, Rue licked the wound, Byron punched Rue, Rue yelped, Byron wrestled him to the ground, Rue rolled over on him, Byron rolled over on Rue, and they got up best friends.

It all went back to a problem with anger. Anger has to do with dominance and dominance has to do with power and as our American forefathers knew, power can lead to abuse, and when you get abused, of course, you get really angry.

The point was, Carter and I needed to awaken our dog-mind. We needed to find our places in the pack. Carter needed to learn how to submit, and I needed to learn how to fight. I did not need, as some psychologists say, to free my "inner child." My inner child generally whimpered and cringed and wanted to be loved. Nor did I need to free my inner male. My inner male (in the interests of sexual parity) also whimpered and cringed and wanted to be loved. I was going deeper than that. What I was attempting to do was to free my inner dog. The dog-mind in the human mind is the master of all domination. The dog-mind does not fear confrontation. The dog-mind seeks power. The dog-mind asserts dominance. But the dog-mind also knows when to quickly tuck the tail between the legs and crouch. The dog-mind knows when to roll over and play dead. The dog-mind doesn't want to kill. It doesn't even need to win. The dog-mind just wants to know where it stands. The dog-mind does not breed resentment and low self-esteem and drug-addiction. The dog-mind does not become enslaved to a substance. The dog-mind knows when to snap and knows when to lick. The dog-mind lets you rise up friends with your enemy. The dog-mind informs you about how to live as a part of the pack, a dog among dogs, a human among humans.

That night, emboldened by my pugnacious success with my students,

I finally called Carter. The Theory of Dog Mind was my answer for Carter. I was thinking any minute I was going to kick butt. Or at least nip gluteus maximus. I was ready for confrontation. My dog-mind was ready. "Carter," I said, "how you doing?"

"Oh, I'm fine," he said in a cheery voice.

In a heartbeat, my resolve crumbled. How could I make him feel bad when he was feeling so cheerful? What did I say now? Gee, Carter, I heard you were on the edge of death?

"Uh, thanks for the e-mail card," I said, referring to the thank-you card he sent via e-mail a few weeks after he got the birthday card I sent him via e-mail.

"Oh, yeah, did you get that?" he said brightly.

We discussed the pros and cons of e-mail cards. We discussed the pros and cons of birthdays. I was getting depressed. When was I going to kick him in the butt with my total honesty? Not now, evidently. My dog-mind was napping.

"Oh," Carter continued, "and please tell Sean that I'm sorry but I can't go to the guitar show at the Museum of Fine Arts." Carter had said he would go with Sean, but he was not doing well enough to go right now.

There it was! My opening. I leaped. "Yeah, I heard from Mom you're having trouble getting around." I didn't mention our sister's anxious call. Carter bristled when Caroline made anxious phone calls. The more anxious Caroline gets, the more she gives advice. Carter thought she was trying to control him. Which, of course, she was. *Somebody* needed to be in control, right?

Now Carter began to talk about his condition as if he had never said "I'm fine" five minutes ago, as if I had been asking a different question altogether then. He breezed on in a cheery voice. I couldn't understand why he didn't sound upset. It was almost as if he *liked* being sick.

"I can't do too much at a time," he said. "I went out to get a hair cut and do the grocery shopping, and I got really sick." Lyndsey had to help him put on his blood-pressure support socks. He couldn't shower often, because he couldn't get dressed by himself. He couldn't take a bath because once he sat down, he couldn't stand up by himself. He was sleeping sitting up because there was fluid around his lungs.

"I feel terrible about this, Carter," I said. "I'm very upset about the condition you're in."

"I know," said Carter. "I feel terrible about it also."

"Are you going to try, you know, another diet?" I asked timidly. My inner dog growled.

"Yeah, I am. I'm going to go back on the Systems House diet. I've just got to get it set up on my computer."

"Oh, that's good, that's really great, Carter." I was ecstatic that he was going to try again. Maybe I wouldn't have to kick his butt after all.

"But it's really important to have some support," he continued. "I'm worried that I won't be able to maintain it. I don't really have any support system."

He had given me the perfect opening. "Well, you can go to OA, Carter. OA would be perfect for you. That's just what it is, a support system." I am all for Overeaters Anonymous, since it is based upon the principles of AA and Al-Anon, which have already helped our family.

"Oh, no," said Carter, "OA is terrible."

My heart sank. "Terrible? What do you mean?"

"Uh," he grunted in disgust. "They're totally not supportive."

I couldn't imagine why Carter was hostile toward OA, but I could hear the edge in his voice. Land mine! I didn't want to lose him altogether, and I dropped the point.

"Well," I burbled on, "maybe the family can be your support system. You can call me. I should go on a diet, too."

Now, anybody who knows anything about family addiction would immediately hear bells clanging and smell the smoke rising. I would be his "support system?" I would go on a diet? How could Carter possibly learn to be a dog among dogs in the tiny circle of his devoted familiars? I had just committed a cardinal Al-Anon sin, an error of magnificent proportion. It is called *"Trying to fix the addict."* In truth, you can only help an addict fix himself. All sorts of alarms were clanging in my head, but I silenced them. *Screw it,* I thought, *it's someplace to start.* I did want to lose some weight anyway.

But then, something really nice happened. There was a pause on the other end of the line.

"Thanks, Cete," said Carter, using my old, baby nickname. His voice sounded funny. Choked up, sort of.

All my defenses immediately collapsed. He knew that I knew that he needed help, and he was grateful that I cared. He wasn't *always* a jerkaholic, after all. In fact, sometimes he was pretty terrific.

"Well," I said, "I love you, Carter." And then the love did come rinsing through my heart, like a painful, white, sulphurous burn, a salt wave from childhood that was scudded with understanding, stinging my nose, aching my throat, staining my eyes.

"I love you, too, Cete," he said.

SEVEN: THERE MUST BE SOMETHING BETTER THAN THIS, 1966 – 1970

*A*BOVE all, I do not want to die.

Dad is always nasty drunk, and Mom is always angry. In the fall of my fourteenth year, I stand in the shower, hot water pounding on my head and back. I make it pound harder, as if it might hammer me into something else. We live in Connecticut now, as strange and foreign a place as Canada. I miss my Long Island friends. The girls at my new junior high school do not like to read or study; they do not like sports; they do not like me.

In school, in the auditorium, Principal Davis drones on about school spirit. Around me, girls are giggling. They are laughing at the boy seated in the row ahead of us. The boy tries to inch his hands back into the loose cuffs of his long-sleeved shirt. Both of his wrists are wrapped round and round with white gauze and tape. The girls whisper that he tried to kill himself.

The girls in this school are idiots. What do they know? They know nothing. How can they laugh at a boy who tried to kill himself?

What I know is this: I want to live.

*   *   *

Carter is applying for a CO. He does not want to go to Vietnam; he is a Conscientious Objector. He would rather move to Canada than fight in Vietnam. I believe the war is wrong, though I do not understand geography, or politics, or power. My objection is simple. I think people shouldn't murder each other.

Carter is a pacifist. After he returned from the Peace Corps, Carter went back to college and switched from Engineering to Sociology. When he graduated, he stayed on in Ithaca to help migrant farm workers. He was even investigated by the FBI because of anti-war protests. Then he got a bad number in the draft lottery.

There is a committee Carter must convince. We drive by the building in which he will have the Conscientious Objector hearing. He rants on and on about how the war is wrong, and I listen politely. He has become a stranger to me, an adult in some faraway land.

What will happen if Carter moves to Canada and can never come home again?

From the car, I can see nothing but concrete and blank windows, and I imagine the faceless committee who will decide if my brother lives or dies. I wonder if he is afraid. I do not understand. How can they order someone who has served in the Peace Corps to go murder people in Vietnam?

But Carter does not have to go to Canada; he does not have to go to Vietnam, either. Nor does he get the status of Conscientious Objector. He qualifies 4F because of high blood pressure. The army doesn't want him.

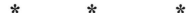

Caroline invites me to visit her in Philadelphia, where she is teaching. I tell her how it is with Mom and Dad, how I have no friends. We talk for hours. No adult has ever listened to me before. Caroline makes me feel smart and special. I throw all my life-lines onto Caroline's boat. I call Caroline; I visit Caroline. She is always there for me. One day at a time, Caroline is saving my life.

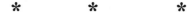

Carter is teaching me to play the guitar. It is the first time we have ever done anything together. He is very patient, and shows me all the chords and picking to play my favorite song. For Christmas, Carter gives me a beautiful, mahogany acoustic guitar, even though I know he does not have any money. I guess Carter likes me after all. *Blue is the color of my true love's eyes,* I sing. I have never had a date, much less a true love. I write songs and ache to be touched.

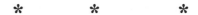

There is a black and white picture of Carter building bathhouses in the Peace Corps. In this picture, he is about a hundred pounds thinner than I've ever seen him. I am amazed by how handsome he looks. His chin and his cheekbones are sharply delineated, and his body is trim in a white shirt and slacks. I guess he made up for lost weight as soon as he returned to America, because now he looks the same as he ever did. I figure he must have lost the weight because he got really sick in Iran. He was in the hospital for a long time with a staph infection and dysentery. Also, he says, the food was terrible.

I have never thought of Carter as handsome, and it seems a shame that he can't lose the weight to look this good again. Not that I would mention it to him; we don't talk about things like that.

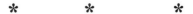

My parents are snickering. Carter is trying to be a coffeehouse guitar player. We are going to a party he is having at his huge commune apartment on the upper West Side in New York City.

From Connecticut, we drive through the darkness on the Merritt Parkway. I stare into the silent landscape from the back seat. In the city, Carter greets my parents eagerly and introduces them to his friends. I wonder why he wants his friends to meet his little sister and his parents. If I had friends, I would have no interest in having them meet Carter or my parents.

Some of the commune members perform in the living room after dinner. Carter dances with his girlfriend, Debbie. His big, heavy body bends awkwardly, and as he reaches toward the sky with one hand and hops precariously on one foot, Debbie vocalizes some bird-like noises. I close my eyes and try not to cringe. My father, who danced with Martha Graham at the beginning of his acting career, is sitting on the floor watching respectfully. Carter plays a few songs on his guitar and sings, as well. That is better, but he goes off-key from time to time. My father and mother clap their hands enthusiastically at the end and shout

"Bravo!" I think they should tell Carter to go back to engineering.

In the car, going home, they shake their heads and laugh. They admire Carter's courage. They marvel at his commune. They cannot understand why in the world he wants to be a singer.

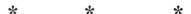

Caroline marries a man from Sweden and moves to Stockholm, where she has a baby girl, Emma. Carter finally quits trying to be a singer and moves to California. Can he get any further away from his family? If he could, he probably would.

I write Caroline long letters, but I hardly communicate with Carter. We aren't sure how he makes a living in San Francisco. He does house cleaning. He works in construction. He has abandoned singing, but he has a new ambition. He is trying to create a new kind of urban commune, something to do with architecture and love and sharing. He works for a while with the innovative architect Solari. He sends home Solari cow bells that hang in the living room.

I do not understand what it is all about. Nor do our parents. When I visit Caroline in Sweden, she says Carter disapproves of the contemporary urban-suburban sprawl, which makes people disenfranchised, and he is trying to build a kind of lifestyle and architecture that will make everyone feel interconnected. But we still don't get it. My parents laugh and shake their heads. Carter has become a joke to them, a special and beloved joke, but a joke nonetheless.

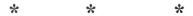

I can hear Mom and Pop screaming at each other in the living room. Pop must be drunk again. The front door slams, and I hear footsteps crunching on the gravel. I hurry to my bedroom window and look out into the dark. It is Mom, leaving. She gets into the car and revs the motor angrily, then drives off.

There is no lock on my door. Pop is stomping around the house. What will happen? I am terrified. My heart is pounding and my hands shake. I curl up on my bed. Sometimes he bursts into my room and starts yelling at me in his deep, gravelly voice, the voice of venom and hatred, telling me to do this or that, telling me I'm bad. Or will he do something even worse … something unmentionable? Who knows? He could do anything when he is drunk.

The other side of my bedroom has a door to the outside. Very quietly, I creep to the door and pull it open. I will hide outside in the bushes until Mom comes back. But what if he comes looking for me? Will he be even more angry if I am hiding? I freeze at the door, uncertain.

From the living room, there is another door slam. A crunching on the gravel. Another car drives off. He is gone. I stagger back to my bed and collapse, the sweat soaking my pajamas. I am safe.

*   *   *

Dune by Frank Herbert is the most amazing book I have ever read, which makes Mom snicker. Try *The Bear* by Faulkner, she suggests, but I find it tedious. This is because I am just not smart enough. Caroline, who has a genius IQ, says smart people like to read science fiction, but I doubt it. Carter doesn't talk about books; he usually talks about getting in touch with your anger. Mom admires Faulkner, Shakespeare, Conrad, James Joyce. Pop admires my poetry. He will sit for hours memorizing my poems; he will talk to me about structure and images. Mom thinks it's great that I write, but she admires *geniuses*: Albert Einstein, Albert Schweitzer, T.S. Eliot, Pound. I gnash my teeth and try to read *The Dry Salvages*. O, I cry into my pillow at night, I will *never* be smart enough.

*   *   *

My father hides his liquor in all kinds of weird places. Once I find a pint of Smirnov in my rubber boot. I never see him drink, but I always know when he is drunk. His eyes get thick and mean. I have two fathers, the drunk and the sober. Sober, he is a different person. He would never say and do all those terrible things to me sober. Would he?

Mom finds Al-Anon, the organization for families of alcoholics, and there is less fighting. Occasionally, Dad tries to get sober. Carter and Caroline don't even believe Dad is an alcoholic. They don't really understand the two fathers. In the living room, the sober father sits in the rocking chair, smoke wreathing his thick, yellowing fingers and black hair. He inhales deeply, blows it out, listening to Mahler in the afternoon gloom. "I guess I'm just not good enough," he says. He thinks he is a failure.

I understand how he feels. There are times when life is almost too painful to bear. Sometimes, it seems, the only good things in life are Ring Dings and science fiction.

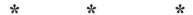

Carter visits from California and lectures me about EST. Werner Erhardt founded EST and Carter is a student and advocate. EST is the answer. EST seminars will cure unhappiness, says Carter. I think Carter is nuts. He's been taken over by commercial zombie fanatics. He presses EST tapes on me. He tries to get my mother and father to listen to EST. Mom and Dad listen and nod and take his tapes, which gather dust in a drawer. I hide in my room and bury myself in *Stranger in a Strange Land*.

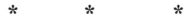

Change or die.

On the New Haven Railroad, tall men in dark suits with dark briefcases pack themselves into the early train headed for New York City. The wind whips the long, cement platform as I push into the stuffy car amongst them. They look askance at the young girl who does not fit, and I rejoice. I am headed for liberty, anonymity, the chance to begin again,

I am going to become a new person. Only I can't do it in Connecticut. Mom thinks we can't afford a private school in Manhattan, but Pop understands. He knows what it is to be an outsider. At the new school, I am going to become a new person: a person with friends, a person who laughs and is confident.

I will change. I will make things better. I refuse to go the other way.

*   *   *

Annie, my new friend from my new school, is sleeping in the other bed. From Annie's apartment bedroom in the Bronx, I can see the long slope of lights on the George Washington Bridge in the night, a white string curving to the red tip like a giant woman's breast.

It is the middle of the night, and I am on the telephone with a hospital emergency room. *"Do you want us to send an ambulance?"*

Miss Melvin, our beloved science teacher who introduced us to the mysteries of psychology and cosmology along with biology, has suggested to me that I might try seeing a psychiatrist. I have dropped to 96 pounds, though I am not anorexic. I just feel nauseous all the time. I can swallow milk. Mom makes health drinks for me in the morning: milk, raw egg, a little sugar and vanilla. She cooks my favorite meals but I can barely eat. "Eat," Mom urges with an anxious look. "You have to eat."

I think perhaps I have a serious illness. I wake up in the dark, terrified. My heart pounds like a runaway train. I press my hand to my neck to take my pulse, then jump out of bed, gasping. How can a heart go so fast? *I'm going to have a heart attack,* I think. *I must have food poisoning.* In a sweat, I call the emergency room of the hosptial.

"Do you want us to send an ambulance?" they ask again.

"No," I say, collapsing to Annie's chair as my heart slows. "No, I'm all right." Even as I speak, my heart slows to normal. I hang up the phone to the emergency room. There is something very wrong with me, but I don't know what it is.

"What is it?" whispers Annie, waking in the other bed.

"I'm okay now," I pant, trembling as she gets out of bed and puts an arm around me.

In the day, it comes on slower, and only when I am alone. The attack begins with a sensation of strangeness. The air seems distant and too loud. Then my flesh begins to feel flattened out and my tongue goes tinny. My heart starts pounding and adrenaline shoots through my veins. *I must have eaten something poisonous. I have food poisoning.* There is an awareness of my hands; as I look at them, it seems they could belong to someone else. *I am going crazy,* I think. *I'm going to have a heart attack.*

Annie finds a catalog of my symptoms in Karen Horney's *Neurotic*

Personality of Our Time. Even the part about thinking I'm having a heart attack. "You're not going crazy," says Annie. "You have an Anxiety Neurosis. Talk to Miss Melvin about it."

"Who is this teacher, anyway!" Mom says to me angrily. She does not want me to go to a psychiatrist. Carter and Caroline think psychiatrists are self-indulgent. But I insist. I fight for it. I do *not* want to die. One brush with death was enough for me. I want to live. My childhood recoils and surges like a distant dream. I am sure there must be something better than this.

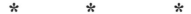

On the hill behind my parents' house, in the woods, Carter – visiting from California – is building a sweat lodge. It is a round hut made of branches tied together and covered with black plastic tarps. Outside, there is a fire pit where he will heat stones. He does some ritual stuff and burns herbs. He will take the hot stones inside and pour water over them. Then all the people will sweat and become pure.

I think that's how it works, anyway. I am not sure, because I don't participate. My parents participate, as do others that Carter invites. Not Caroline; Caroline is still in Stockholm, working at a Peace Research Institute and taking care of her new baby, Emma. She wouldn't have come anyway; she's too intellectual. Demonstrations of emotional and religious fervor embarrass her.

Carter shakes his medicine bag and recites complicated rituals he learned from an American Indian medicine man in Arizona, where they named him Bear. They gave Carter a Native American name, but they would not accept him into their tribe. He is, after all, not Native American. In fact, I think one of our pre-Revolutionary forebears tracked Native Americans. How can you get more Anglo-Saxon than that?

I am annoyed by the whole thing. Sweating just gives me a migraine, anyway. Use a water filter if you want purity!

Why doesn't he just go to church like a good Protestant if he wants religion? Not only does Carter-Bear spend the day chanting, he has also stolen my only copy of *Black Elk Speaks*. Why does he pretend to be something that he is not? Everyone in our family is pretentious. What a jerkaholic, I think, and I drive myself to my psychiatrist appointment. I do not like my psychiatrist, but he's all I've got. He says I have had only bad experiences with men and I feel that my mother doesn't love me. That's ridiculous, I say. Of course my mother loves me. I just want to know why I keep dreaming that aliens have invaded the earth and I am too late to save my family from death.

EIGHT: DOCTOR SORRY
March

*I*T was 9 a.m., two weeks after the initiation of crisis mode in Operation Carter. In the kitchen, dishes were collecting in the sink. On the counter, the backpack papers, the books, the spelling tests, the B&B messages, the peanut butter and jelly jars, the credit card solicitations, the catalogues, the spotting bananas, the newspapers, and the Dorito chips were already backing up. The hateful message machine was blinking like a Cyclops. On the linoleum floor was a splotch of indeterminate brownish stuff and one very hunky, unfurling rawhide dog bone originally shaped to resemble a turkey-leg.

A couple of Carter's doctors called back, but I had missed their calls. I scratched Rue's ears with my toes while I dialed all of Carter's doctors again.

"Well, when *can* I speak to Doctor Mumblejumble?" I repeated sternly to the receptionist of my brother's illustrious cardiac surgeon.

"Mumble mumble *mumble* busy," said the receptionist. "Mumble emergency mumble mumble."

"Well, can I speak to the nurse?"

"Mumble mumble call you back?" said the receptionist.

I agreed with a surly tone. How could I possibly make progress here? I might have to do something else, like wash the floor. My anxiety mounted.

Then the pulmonary specialist called back. He was gruff and jolly, and I imagined him to have sparkling eyes and a big brown beard, like Santa Claus when he was young.

"What a *good* sister you are!" he raved. "Carter really needs his family in there pitching for him."

O most excellent surgeon, I thought. *O most salutary doctor!* No wonder my brother loved this guy. "Oh, I don't know if I can really make a difference," I answered modestly.

"If he can lose just a little of the weight," said the pulmonary specialist, "if he can just lose 20 or 30 or maybe 50 pounds, it will help him a great deal. His heart just isn't strong enough to pump the blood around. The fluid starts to pool around his lungs. That's why he's having so much trouble breathing. If he loses some of the weight, his heart won't have to work so hard and the fluid won't build up like that."

I hung up from this call feeling elated. I made an energetic round of call-backs to all of the other doctors and left second messages. As I was doing this, Carter's former cardiac specialist, the one who was too far away for Carter to see very often, called back.

"How is Carter doing?" said a soft, sweet voice, heavily accented with what sounded like an Indian dialect.

"Not very well," I said. "He's over 400 pounds now, and he's having trouble walking around."

"Oh, my," said the doctor. "I am very sorry to hear that."

The funny thing was, I believed that he was indeed very sorry, and his very sorriness squeezed up next to my heart and made me feel like I was going to cry again.

"I want to see if I can help him in any way," I said, clearing my throat and trying to keep the tremble out of my voice.

"Can he go back to the Systems House program, where was it, in Virginia? I think he lost quite a bit of weight there before, didn't he?"

"It sounds like he can't. I think he is too sick to go back there. His condition is too fragile."

"Yes," said Doctor Sorry. "It's too bad. Most of the people who go away to those places gain the weight back after they come home. I'm not sure how effective it is, anyway."

"I don't know what to do. Will it help him at this point to lose weight? Would it help his heart condition? Could he get rid of the diabetes? The pulmonary doctor said it would be good if he lost even a little weight."

"Oh, yes," said the doctor. "It will lessen the stress on his heart if he can lose some weight. I don't think the diabetes will ever go away now, but he could manage it with less insulin, and that would be a good thing. But it will definitely lessen the stress on his heart if he can lose some weight."

"Well, how can I get him to lose some weight?"

"I don't know," said Doctor Sorry sadly.

There was an awkward silence. "Well, thank you very much for your call, Doctor," I said.

"Please. Call me any time. I'm glad to help."

And he really was, too. Isn't it funny how some people are so kind and caring and some are not? Why is that? When Carter was a teenager, why did he fail to find the people in life who were caring? Why did he get beaten down by the people who were unkind? In my exercise class, for example, four out of the six other women were not kind. They were cool. They were hip. They were bone! They were brand new Nikes and pulled back hair. They were friends with the teacher and knew each others' names. Their eyes slid past me like sunlight gliding over the Hudson River. I was as blank to them as cold water on a winter day.

"What you don't understand," said Doreen when I discussed my exercise-class social problems with her, "is that some people just don't *care* if you like them. They don't *want* to connect with you. They don't *want* to be your friend. It doesn't matter to them. They have other ways of feeling good about themselves."

My jaw dropped in dumb surprise. This was an entirely new concept to me. These people didn't care what I thought? They didn't *want* my friendship? She was right. I did not understand. Here was the seat of a certain power that I had never considered. The power of not caring. How did they do it? How could you possibly be in a class with somebody, sweating and hopping and tilting your pelvis and kicking your legs together week after week, and never care enough to say good morning or even make eye contact? How could you be so self-sufficient?

This was a very foreign land, a new country, a mysterious far-stretching field where people felt good in a manner that had nothing to do with loving or being loved. I tiptoed in to take a look. What was it, what was it? Their thrones were turned away.

Of course, I reasoned, they must care about being loved by *somebody*. They just didn't care about connecting with *me*.

And then it hit me. An awesome revelation: They thought I was unimportant!

Moi, *unimportant*? How could they be so stupid? Of course, if you looked at it from their point of view, I *was* a completely obscure, slightly overweight, rather short, middle-aged mother hopping around tilting her pelvis to a sanitized aerobic version of Norwegian Wood, but that was no reason to think I was unimportant. For all they knew, I could be a compassionate, witty, sensitive poet in disguise.

If I were, say, a famous writer, I thought resentfully, or a movie star, or even a prospective client for business, then I would be important, I bet! Then they'd want to be my friend. And, maybe, if I were very cool like them, they might *suspect* I was important, and then they'd want to be my friend, too. Just in case.

Okay, I thought. I knew these people. I'd met these people before. People like this stridently advocate today's most popular brand of tolerance while cutting a neighbor because she lives in a trailer. They judge according to the preferred list of criteria. Why didn't they approach people like dogs, sniffing and tail-wagging until they figured out whether a person deserved to be growled at or licked? Because they didn't trust themselves, that's why; they had no center; they had no dog-mind. Poor things, they believed they were superior to dogs, when in reality, they were functioning on the level of sheep.

Did I still want these dolts to like me? Of course I did. The difference was, now I knew I shouldn't.

"What a bunch of jerks," I said to Doreen. "Who cares if they're unfriendly!"

"Yeah, who cares!" cheered Doreen, knowing full well that I did.

"You gotta toughen up," Sean always said. "You gotta climb into that rhino skin." Sean was abandoned by his alcoholic Village-Beatnik mother when he was a baby, so he has had a lot of time to practice.

Somehow, the folks in my family just did not develop a strong hide. All of us were extremely sensitive to rejection. We felt every lump that came our way, right down to the heart. "Oversensitive in the extreme …" said Bill Wilson in his analysis of the alcoholic personality. How would my brother have fared if he had developed some rhinohide?

I plugged in my laptop and jumped onto the Internet to find the answers for my brother. I input "food addiction" on my primary search engine. No results. I input "compulsive over-eating." Ah, 242 hits. Hey, hadn't I done that before with no results at all? I must have spelled it differently. Web sites advertised psychologists, diet books, diet programs, and self-help groups for the sexually abused. Medical sites yielded long and branching avenues of information: "Bariatrics," I learned, is the branch of medicine that deals with obesity.

But I did not find one rehabilitation center for compulsive overeating. Where could a person go if he needed to remove himself from food, food, food, and recover from food-addiction?

I input the word *rehab*. I got 272,668 websites. The first 100 were for drug and alcohol rehabilitation or physical rehabilitation. Nothing for compulsive overeating.

How about *"rehab for compulsive overeaters"*? My search produced no results. Not one. I went to *Ask Jeeves*. Where could I find a rehab for compulsive over-eaters? Now I got lots of answers, but most of them just defined compulsive over-eating and offered self-help programs. Then, hosannas, I found something: The Center for Eating Disorders. *They treated compulsive over-eaters.* And they even had an inpatient hospital program for people who were already very sick! The web site said the Center was one of the few that existed, and by now, I believed it.

Eagerly, I searched the site. Most insurance covered treatment, they said. I was surprised. The health insurance did not pay for Carter's stay at Systems House – Mom did.

Did the Center have a good support program for when you went home? There was no point in it if there was no support after the rehab. We already knew from Carter's previous experience at Systems House that even when he lost weight and ate right while he was there, he fell back into his old patterns as soon as he got home. Then he gave up hope and didn't even try. I found the answer: Yes, the Center did offer relapse-prevention and organized eating-disorder support groups for after you went home. O, rapture! This was, perhaps, The Answer.

Suddenly, I realized I had not seen a real-world address. My heart sank. Where was this place, anyway? After a thorough search of the web site, I found an actual, land-based address: Palo Alto.

California?

Failure descended like a mortar shell. No way Carter would go so far away from Lyndsey, and we could never afford to house Lyndsey in California with Carter. Anyway, she couldn't afford to leave her job. I thought he would be afraid to leave his doctors in Massachusetts, too. Plus, he would have no support program after he got out.

I was exhausted and disappointed. It was 3:25. I had a headache and realized I had not eaten all day.

Then, suddenly, something else hit me: I had forgotten to pick the children up from school.

Springing out of my chair, I lunged for my coat and tripped over the mass of wires pooled at my feet. The modem pulled out and I managed to catch the laptop as it slid off the table. Suddenly, the phone rang. My feet were still snarled in the modem wire, and I knocked the telephone receiver to the floor. A little but loud voice boomed up at me from the linoleum.

"Mommy? Mommy, where are you?"

I knelt and put my head against the phone. "Harry?"

"Mommy! Where are you?"

Where was I? In truth, that was hard to say. On the floor? On the Internet? In the kitchen? With Carter? Inside my head? I was rarely in just one place. "I'm coming," I said.

"We're *waiting*!" Harry said indignantly. "The phone was busy for *hours*! We've been waiting in the office for almost – almost – a whole hour."

"Two hours," I heard his younger brother chime in from the background.

"Get out of here, Byron."

I could see Harry pushing Byron off, keeping control of the electronics. Over the line, I heard the office secretary scolding them. In reality, I was only fifteen minutes late, but that was enough to inconvenience everyone in the whole school.

"I'm coming," I said, and rushed out the door.

In the principal's office, Mrs. Marsh, the secretary, greeted me with cold eyes and pursed lips. We both looked at the clock. I was 22 minutes late. The children jumped on me and started telling me about recess, their favorite subject.

"I'm terribly sorry, Mrs. Marsh," I said to the secretary. "I lost track of the time."

"*Hrrumph, pumph, pumppump,*" said Mrs. Marsh, getting on her coat and avoiding my eyes.

"I'm so sorry I made you stay late," I said desperately, staggering as Byron pogoed on my arm to beat out Harry at who could command my attention first. "Stop it!" I growled, shaking them off. They dropped their backpacks and raced out the front door.

Mrs. Marsh threw me a bone. "*Hrumph, pumph,* had to stay anyway," she conceded, shutting down her computer.

She hated me, I knew, and not just because I did things like forget my children, but more because I had this irritating tendency to break the rules. I got impatient and I was always rushing around and I sometimes tried to sneak around rules, and I *always* got caught. "*Who was that?*" they would squawk over the walkie talkie as I snuck by the office to pick up my kids without queuing on the interminable car-line. "*It's Mrs. S—.*" They used my married name at school. "*Mrs. S—?*" "*Yes, Mrs. S—.*" The walkie-talkie static would come at me from both directions as I scurried along the hall. "*Where's she going?*" "*I don't know. To the gym?*" "*The gym?*" "*She didn't sign in.*" "*Where is she?*" "*She didn't sign in?*" "*Here she is. She's in the gym.*" I was like a bad odor wafting through a low-budget movie.

I signed the children out with chastened and lowered eyes. Would Mrs. Marsh be nice to me if I obeyed all the rules? Probably. But then *I* might hate *her*.

I have decided that one of the terrible things about life is that it is simply impossible to make everybody love you. No matter what you do, somebody hates you. Even if you do nothing, somebody doesn't like you for that! For example, after picking up the kids late, I pulled into the gas station to just get a newspaper and a snack for the kids, and (my heart swelling with consideration for my fellow man) I did *not* park at the busy pumps, where it would have been easy to ditch the car for a minute, but pulled into the last, tight, parking space next to the deli, where somebody had sliced off half the spot by parking crooked. As I squeezed out of the passenger side, my door gently kissed the car next to me (not the one parked crookedly, the one on the other side). I saw the woman in the driver's seat, her window rolled up, jerk her head as her eyes flicked toward the back of her car. Then she gazed at the worm that used to be me.

I smiled and waved reassuringly at her. "It's not hurt!"

She muttered something ferocious into her steaming coffee cup. She looked right at me. I couldn't hear what she was saying, but I could tell it was nasty.

I stopped in front of her window and grinned my most terrifying grin. My dog-mind was yapping. "Excuse me?" I said in a loud voice, peering at her through the glass. *You wanna say that to my face?*

She did. She rolled her window down. She did not appear to be terrified. Her large, hazel eyes were as hard and crackling as frozen milk, the soft skin tight with indignation. "Your response is inappropriate!"

"But I didn't hurt it," I said. "I just touched it."

"You should apologize!"

I was nonplussed. I thought maybe she really didn't understand. "But I … I didn't *hit* it, it just…." I was about to demonstrate how my car door just gently *leaned* on her car so I could squeeze out and as I did so, I almost touched her car *again*. Quickly, I caught myself and demonstrated how gentle I was on my own car. "I just *touched* it, like this."

But the drums of war were beating. "Your response is inappropriate," she said angrily. "You should apologize!"

I growled, my heart pounding, and stalked into the deli, which had already run out of my newspaper. I bought a whole box of chocolate Ring Dings and ate three on the spot. By the time I got back out, the crooked car was gone and I was able to get into my car on the driver's side. The mean lady on the other side and I did not look at each other.

"No good deed goes unpunished," Sean always says. I felt terrible. The family illness reared its ugly head. I thought how I should have apologized to the lady, how I should have waited in line at school, what a jerk I was, and how I was never, *ever* going to try to be helpful ever again. How could that lady not know that I was a nice person who really cared about being good? Or was it that she could see the *real* me, that me that was hidden even to myself, and the *real me* actually *was* a bad person, a person who laughed and was careless and touched other people's cars?

The dark night of the soul overtook my afternoon. I screamed at my kids for making a mess in the back seat with Yodels and Ring Dings. If I was bad, they must be bad, too! They looked scared. Two minutes later, I pulled the car over and apologized for losing my temper at them. I told them they were good and wonderful, that I was feeling kind of down today and it made me lose my temper, even though they really *should* throw their garbage in the garbage bag and the car really was shamefully filthy. I keep hoping if I tell them I am wrong, if I let them know when I rage at them it is because there is something wrong with me, they won't get as crazy as I am. Please be less crazy than my family, boys, because I love you so much. Please be happy and well-adjusted and normal even though you come from the visible body of my spiritually bankrupt family.

Once, I thought just as my father did: If you got famous, if you became a movie star, then everybody would love you and you could be happy. Man, *nobody* would yell at you for touching their car. They'd ask you to sign your name in its dust! That's what my father wanted; he wanted to be a movie star so everybody would love him and think how wonderful he was and nobody would ever hurt his feelings or make him feel bad about himself again. Ha! Little did he know until he became a TV matinee idol that if half the people love you when you're famous, the other half hate you for it. How can you win? You can't!

I ate another three Ring Dings on the way home and decided to call Carter.

"Carter," I said to him, "did you know that *I* have an eating problem also? Did I ever tell you about that?"

"Really?" said Carter.

"Yes," I said. "In fact, in college, I became a failed bulimic. Didn't I ever tell you about that?"

"No," said Carter, fascinated. We had never really discussed our mutual disorders.

"Yeah, I would binge and binge on sweets till I was sick. Then I would try to throw up, but I couldn't. Don't you remember I gained about 25 pounds in six months?"

"No," said Carter. Since I had been so underweight when I went to college, because of my high-school panic disorder, the extra weight hadn't been that noticeable.

"Yeah, and now I've been on a diet for twenty years." Sometimes I remembered my panic disorder with a touch of nostalgia.

"Twenty years!" said Carter. "That's almost as bad as me!"

"Yeah," I said eagerly. "I really have a problem with sweets. I try to swear off altogether, but I always slip up."

"You should try this Systems House diet," said Carter. He explained the elaborate diet that had been given to him by the place where he went away to lose weight.

"Yeah, but ..." I said. He didn't hear me. Once Carter got rolling on a subject, he usually kept going until the subject had reached its conclusion. He told me how you determine the calories.

"Yeah, but ..." I said. He didn't hear me again. He explained the way the program worked, the balance, the menu, the work you have to do on the computer.

"I should be doing it myself," he said, "but it's very complicated to set up. I've never set it up on my computer."

Yeah, but ..." I said. He bumped over me like a runaway golf cart.

Now I remembered why I had not shared the details of my problems with him before. However, I tried again. "I don't know if that would work for me. You know why? You know why I think that might not work for me? Carter? You know why?"

"Huh?" said Carter, pulling up short.

"See, I don't think that would work for me because the problem I have is just with sweets – when I eat sweets, I just can't stop. Even diet desserts. If I could just stop eating sweets, you know, I don't think I'd have a problem."

"Oh," he said. He sounded disappointed. Even though Carter did not seem to be able to help himself, he loved to help other people. If you didn't want his help, then his feelings got hurt and he crawled back into his shell again. Now I'd managed to tell him that he couldn't help me, either. And if he couldn't help me, what was he talking about all this for?

There was an awkward pause. I was losing him. Why the heck did I say that? Trying to be honest? Not really. More like I got pissed off that he doesn't listen to me. I could have kicked myself. Anxiously, I tried to think of a way he could help me.

Then I had a sudden and brilliant brainstorm. "But you know," I said, "maybe I would be more successful if I *did* a balanced eating plan like that. Maybe if I ate a balanced diet with the right amount of calories and everything, maybe then I wouldn't have so much trouble quitting sugar."

"Yeah!" Carter said immediately with renewed enthusiasm. "I think it would help you."

"And," I added slyly, "maybe we could, you know, *do it together!*"

This was the key! This was it! Excitement surged. If I could get *him* to go on a diet in order to help *me* diet, maybe he would succeed.

"Yeah," said Carter eagerly. "I can work the whole thing out for you on the computer."

I was on a roll. I could feel it. "That'd be great!" I said. "Once you get it set up, you can work yours out too, right? Then we can do it together."

"I need to know your level of activity," he said, the buttons and levers already moving in his mind. "You input all of your personal statistics like your height and weight ..."

"Yeah, and we'll ..." I unsuccessfully interjected.

"... well, that's the usual stuff, but you also put in all of your usual activities and the program calculates the calories that you usually burn and puts it into the diet ...

"Yeah, and we're gonna do it together, right?"

"... and it takes into consideration your age and gender, like I was telling Mom about it and I'd input for her exercise class three times a week, plus ..."

I was beginning to experience melt-down. "And we're going to do it together, right?" I said.

"I really have to get the program set up," he continued. He took a couple of puffy kinds of breaths, and alarms jingle-jangle in my head. "Mom wants me to work out a diet for her, too." *Puff, puff.*

"Oh, great, that's great," I said. "Are you okay there, Carter?"

"It's really a fantastic program," he said. His breathing was definitely getting labored. It sounded like he was doing sit-ups while he was talking. "The people at Systems House created it. I don't know why more people don't know about it. They should really have a better sales effort or something…"

"Carter, wait a minute. Carter? Carter? Uh, I wanted to ask, do you think we'll do it together? Carter, uh, do you think … Uh, Carter!"

"Huh?" He stopped talking. For a moment, I couldn't remember what I wanted to say. Something about the diet.

"Are you okay?"

"Yeah, I'm fine."

I could hear him breathing. Shallow, tiny, raspy breaths. It reminded me of something. The sound of my firstborn Harry when he was a brand new infant, lying on my chest in the hospital bed, his nose next to my ear, sleeping.

He was waiting. Pressure! I had a window of opportunity here. My mind was numb. Frozen. About the diet. How was I going to put it? Anxious, I stumbled bluntly to the point.

"Are you going to do the diet, too, Carter?"

"Uh," said Carter, as if the thought had just struck him. But the logic of the moment was ineluctable. "Sure."

"Then we can do it together."

"Yeah," he said enthusiastically, taking shallow breaths. "We can do it together."

NINE: MY WILD RHUBARB CRUMBLE
March

*T*HE next morning I woke up with a migraine, which was not surprising since I ate a total of nine Ring Dings, two handfuls of mini mint chocolate-chips, plus half a container of Betty Crocker Extra Fudgy Chocolate Frosting the night before. There was something about the prospect of going on a new diet the next day that made a chocolate celebration with your cooking supplies seem reasonable at ten p.m. the night before. Now I had a chocoholic hangover.

"Mommy," Byron frowned at me, "did you eat bad stuff last night?"

Byron knew very well I ate bad stuff last night, since he and the dog helped me demolish the Betty Crocker Extra Fudgy Chocolate Frosting container. I was dragging around the kitchen with the lights off, waiting for the Imitrix to kick in, trying to make lunches for school with my knuckles grinding into my left temple. Imitrix tended to enable my bad eating habits because it could really handle a migraine. This medication was a fabulous new invention that, unlike painkillers, actually stopped a migraine cold. It didn't make you high and carried only minimal risk of your dropping dead from a heart attack or a brain embolism. Migraine sufferers could shoot up Imitrix and get instant relief, but I felt that if you suffered a little more, the risk of your brain exploding lessened, so I popped the pill form, which took at least an hour to kick in.

"Byron," snapped Harry, "don't be rude. Mommy doesn't feel well."

"I *know* Mommy doesn't feel well," Byron retorted indignantly. "I'm trying to help."

"Well, you're not being helpful by being rude."

"I'm not being rude, you're being rude."

"I'm not being rude, *you're* being rude."

There was a sound of feet swinging under the breakfast table. I tried to hide under the hood of the stove.

"Maaaaaaa, he *kicked* me," wailed Byron.

"You kicked me first," shouted Harry.

I pressed both hands into my head. "Stop it, stop it, boys. I have a *headache*."

"He started it," said Byron, grabbing the sugar bowl under cover of full riot gear.

"Mommy, he's putting *sugar* on his Rice Crispies. Mommy! *Mommy!*" Harry was screaming with hysterical, Hitlerian fervor. *"Stop it, Byron. You're not allowed to have sugar."* I heard the sugar bowl being dragged back and forth across the table. Rue barked and there was a bump and a crunchy, scuffley sound amidst the shrieks. I risked a look under my arm and glimpsed little sneakers swinging above the dog, who was eagerly licking sugar off the floor.

I was going to kill somebody soon, and I tried to think of alternatives. Take the dog for a walk? Too cold. Hide in pantry closet? Too cramped. I knew. *Get back in bed.* That sounded like a really good one. Both warm *and* effective!

I trotted past the children with both hands helmeting my head.

"If you don't stop it now and clean up this mess, you will both have to eat *school lunch*."

The silence was instantaneous.

I dove into bed and appropriated the covers off Sean, who had been laid off from his union job the day before and was taking his new status literally. "Honey," I said, "you gotta take the kids to school. I've got a terrible migraine."

"Mmmm," he groaned. "Okay." He started snoring again.

I settled my head into the welcoming feathers of some unhappy goose. Already, the pain was subsiding. A few minutes later, the bedroom door creaked and there was tiptoeing.

"Mommy?" said a little voice.

"Mommy?" said another little voice.

"We'll be good."

Byron tiptoed up in front of me, leaning his face close until his huge, dewy eyes were millimeters from mine. "Do we *really* have to eat school lunch?"

Harry rested against the bed and pressed a cool hand to my forehead. "Do you feel better yet, Mommy?" He added hopefully, "We put Rue outside."

"We put our dishes in the sink!" urged Byron.

It was so lovely to feel needed! I stretched, luxuriating in my moment of power. The rest of the headache drained off. "Are you going to stop fighting? Are you going to be good and kind and love each other like brothers should?"

"Yes!" they pledged in unison, giving each other hugs to demonstrate their seriousness of purpose.

"Then you'll have to ..." I grabbed Byron and threw him on the bed, "... defeat the Tickle Monster first." Harry jumped on top of me and we rolled around tickling each other.

"What's going on?" Sean mumbled sleepily. We tickled him and he rose to his hands and knees, braying like a donkey.

In the end, I bought the boys Lunchables and we were 17 minutes late for school. Consequently, I had to go into the office and fill out two Tardy Excuses, on which I wrote, "Mom sick today," which I felt was an honest if not appropriate excuse. Had I written, "Mom sick every day!" it would have been even more honest, but twenty years of psychotherapy have taught me that total honesty is an obsessive-compulsive disorder. Anyway, self-flagellation did not make you feel better, nor did it make people like you better, so there really was no point to it. Mrs. Marsh, the office secretary, pretended that I was invisible and I chose not to disabuse her of this illusion today. Meekly, I deposited my Tardy Excuses in the Notes Basket and departed.

All day, I was virtuous. I didn't exactly start my new diet, but I didn't eat any more sweets, either. I did all of the work that I was supposed to do, like washing dishes, paying overdue bills, rewashing the laundry that had gone smelly waiting for the dryer, harassing the health insurance to pay up, mopping the floor, finishing the abstract for "Sprains of the Neck Other than Whiplash" (destined for *Judicial Medicine* to help some poor schmo sue some other poor schmo when the health insurance won't pay up), answering B&B e-mail, setting the alarm clock to remind myself to eat lunch before I pick up the children, answering the phone, throwing the laundry into the dryer and folding the dry stuff, calling a developmental psychiatrist to ask for strategies to deal with "Holiday Gimmies" in seven-to-ten year olds for a *FamilyTime* article (my solution, "Slapping Upside the Head," is not an option), stripping the beds, hanging up on telemarketers before they can pick up after I pick up, scribbling an idea about "the dream deferred" into my notebook for later development, running around the house trying to find the beeping smoke alarm only to finally realize that it's the alarm clock and I've forgotten to eat lunch again, picking the children up, making snacks, going to the grocery store and buying a cooked chicken which I partially devour hidden behind the lettuces in the middle of the fruits and vegetables section, calling the car mechanic, searching for the income tax receipts, fixing the dinner, and supervising homework.

Throughout the day, although I did not work obsessively on a poem destined for obscurity, I did fantasize a lot about Thoreau and Walden Pond. O the serenity! O the singleness of purpose! Of course, he didn't have kids, did he! He didn't even have a significant other out there at the pond. Can you imagine the arguments? She wants curtains, he wants natural light. He wants to borrow an ax, she wants to buy. Oh, Henry, it's so easy to simplify when you live alone! But then, well … you're *alone,* aren't you!

The real solution to life, of course, is to win a million dollars. What I would do if I won a million dollars is one of my best fantasies. In fact, I was sitting dreamy-eyed at the table after dinner, my chin on my fists (the children and Sean having escaped into the basement before I could remind them that *we all do the dishes together),* thinking about how much of my million I would apportion to my mortgage and how much to my housekeeper, when the phone rang and Mom's voice – hesitant and apologetic – floated in from the kitchen.

"Uh, I hate to bother you, uh, I know you're very busy," I heard over the answering machine, "but, well, I just thought you should know that Carter's back in the hospital again."

My heart sank into my stomach, where my dinner congealed in a cold lump.

"He's in very good spirits. They don't think he'll be in there too long. I don't know exactly, I think it's his spleen or his pancreas or one of those things – he's been throwing up. He got sick in the night. You know they gave him all that medication when his legs swelled up. I think it's something with the medication; they have to get the medication adjusted or something. Anyway, I'll give you his number, if you just want to get a pencil, maybe you could call him sometime, you know, but his spirits are, you know, good, he seems to be coping very well, and here is the number, it's seven – oh – five – two – two – three ...." Speaking very slowly and enunciating clearly, she followed the telephone number with the number of his room, the address of the hospital, and the telephone number of the nurses' station on his floor, as if the specifics of his place might draw the sting from the uncertainty of his future. "He thinks he won't be in there too long, just until they get his medication adjusted, or somebody gave him the wrong medicine or something, I don't know why they have to pump him up with so much medication for this and medicine for that and nobody seems to know what the other one is doing..." Her voice, lapsing into bitterness, began to quaver and she pulled back to safer topics. "Anyway, you don't have to call him, he's in very good spirits, I know you're very busy, but I just thought you'd want to know ..."

The answering machine, as if sympathetic to Mom's inability to end the message, cut her off.

This persistence of my brother's good spirits was puzzling. For years, he was angry and depressed. Now his body was failing him and he was always in a good mood. He said it was because at last he had someone who really loved him, and it was true that Lyndsey was remarkably kind and loyal, but I found his equanimity strange. Sometimes I wondered if he needed his illness. Perhaps in some way, it took him off the hook; it made him judge himself less harshly. Did he feel more comfortable in life because he was sick?

I called him, and when he picked up the phone, he did sound quite cheerful, just like Mom said.

"They just got me in here for some tests," he said. "They think it's my pancreas."

I had never given the pancreas its fair due. I never knew it could cause so much trouble. In fact, I had never really given my pancreas a second thought. Where was it? What was its function? (Knowing our family, probably something to do with bile.)

"I'm sorry I didn't finish the diet plan for you," he continued. "I was working on it yesterday. I got it about half done."

There was a vague memory in my mind that I had agreed to some kind of diet. "Oh, Carter, don't worry about that! What happened? You seemed to be fine yesterday."

"Well, actually, last night I was having trouble breathing. I'm over here where the pulmonary guy is. He's really a great doctor. He kind of takes the big view. He thinks there's fluid building up around my lungs because of the medication I was taking for the pancreas, because my kidneys weren't flushing it out fast enough, which has to do with my heart not being strong enough to pump it through fast enough…"

As his organs circled in a vast food-chain around my head, devouring each other, what I was thinking was this: Lyndsey once told me, a couple of years ago, that she was pretty sure Carter wasn't really staying on his diet. That she had found pie wrappers in the garbage and had found cookie crumbs on the bedside table. And wasn't that just the picture of my father swigging down his woodshed stash of vodka behind the trees in the back, pulling weeds that turned out to be my patch of wild rhubarb? No more Wild Rhubarb Crumble for me! Lyndsey has told us that Carter shoots up extra insulin just so that he can digest the extra sugar. I didn't know much about the pancreas, but I'd bet that could have a really damaging effect.

I called Lyndsey, The Source, for further information. She didn't sound alarmed. "It's a little difficult to tell. I'm starting to realize Carter doesn't always tell me everything the doctor says."   Yeah, I think, he probably doesn't mention the doctor's instructions such as, *Don't use so much insulin,* and, *You have to lose weight immediately.*

"He doesn't like everybody to get all worried about him, you know?" Lyndsey continued. "He plays it down sometimes. But I don't think this is too bad. I think this is just about his medications. They've got to adjust his medications and they have to make sure he doesn't get pneumonia again. They think he's going to be out tomorrow."

Okay, if he was not going to die right now, this meant The Plan would move ahead. Lyndsey was impressed that I had called all of Carter's doctors and actually heard back from a few.

"They said that even losing a little weight will help him," I told her.

"Yes," she agreed, "I'm sure it would. Maybe he could even get healthy again." She sounded a little wistful, and I got a terrible pang. Poor Lyndsey!

"I'm not sure the diabetes will ever go away," I cautioned her. "They say that it might get a little better, though."

"I'm sure he would feel better if he just ate right."

"See, he really needs a support system, Lyndsey. He can't do this alone. I think that's the real problem."

She got a little defensive. "I just can't be in charge of his eating, CL. He won't listen to me. He just gets angry and says I'm interfering."

Of course, this was exactly like an addict. The illness snarls and spits like a caged animal. It bites any hand that attempts to help it.

"No, that's not what I meant," I assured her. "You can't be his support system. I think we have to get him to go to Overeaters Anonymous."

If we couldn't find a rehab for Carter to go away to, then we had to insist that he begin OA meetings.

"Oh, not OA," Lyndsey said immediately. "He won't go to OA."

"Why not?" I shot back, impatient. I was tired of figuring out perfect solutions that wouldn't work. "We have to *force* him to go to OA!"

"He's already tried OA."

"When did he try OA?"

Lyndsey told me he was going to OA when they met, and how he tried it again near Boston, but hated it.

"I can't believe that OA is not supportive. That's what he said, that it wasn't supportive. How can that be?"

"Oh, yeah, the meeting was terrible. I went with him."

With this news, I was really shocked. I could understand Carter's hostility toward OA. That was the addiction talking. But Lyndsey?

"How could that be?" I asked her. "The whole reason for OA to exist is to be supportive."

"They have what they call these 'gray sheet' meetings," said Lyndsey. "It's like a meal plan and if you don't do the gray sheet, you can't be part of the meeting. All the meetings around here are gray sheet meetings. You know, OA wasn't like that back in Connecticut. Carter was going to do his Systems House diet, but he couldn't do it at OA because of the gray sheet plan."

This sounded incredibly suspicious to me. OA was based upon AA, and AA had only one requirement for membership: a desire to stop drinking. That meant OA should have only one requirement for membership: a desire to stop overeating.

"I don't believe it!" I said to Lyndsey. "That can't be right. That's totally antithetical to the principles of AA."

"It's true," said Lyndsey. "I went to the meetings with him myself. It was really awful."

The heat started to build up behind my ears. This was how I could tell when I was getting mad. The heat began behind my ears, streaked down into my neck like blood poisoning, then sprang up into my cheeks. My heart began to thump.

"That's horrible," I said. "That is bullshit. I can't believe it."

"Yeah, I don't get it, either."

The thing that was really horrible was the fact that my brother actually went for help and didn't get it. He actually acknowledged his addiction, went to OA, and was rebuffed. He might have been headed toward health right now if OA had welcomed him, I think. He might have already gotten better.

Now I was really mad. My whole head was hot. I was sure something was fishy here. "I'm going to investigate this, Lyndsey. I'm sure OA is not supposed to be like that!"

Lyndsey murmured encouraging words that were drowned out by angry screeching from the basement, followed by Sean's hoarse shouts, which sounded a lot like Rue barking. In fact, Rue was barking in the kitchen, too, and I scrambled up from my seat at the still dirty dinner table. *Oh, my God,* I realized with dismay, *it's almost bedtime.* Saying goodbye to Lyndsey, I charged down to the basement and screamed at the boys for fighting. Unfortunately, Sean did not back me up. Sean did not even hear me because he was already back in his music room with the earphones on, shielded by three feet of thick, basement concrete, playing guitar and listening to feedback.

"And," I finished scolding the children with lightning in my eyes and a final shudder of my jowls, *"you didn't help with the dishes!"*

"I cleared my place and washed all my dishes," said Harry, not even glancing up from the mammoth Lego WWII aircraft carrier he was constructing. "And I washed the pot with the corn in it. And I fed Rue. And I put the leftover corn in a Baggie and put it in the fridge."

"Uh," I grunted, my eyes sliding to the upper right corner of my eyelids as if the vague memory of blurred shapes passing by me as I spoke on the phone might resolve themselves into an image of Harry washing dishes.

"Mommy," said Byron, "I am so *exasperated!*"

"Huh?"

"Harry took all of my Lego soccer players and he has them on his aircraft carrier," said Byron.

The issue of the dirty dishes seemed to be getting lost and I was wondering how I could rekindle it.

"He said I could use them." Harry still did not glance up.

"They're not army men, they're soccer players."

"You said I could use them. I let you use my M-17 for your GI Joe."

Byron's voice began to rise again. "I said you could use *one*, not all of them!"

"I said you could use *all* of my M-17s!"

Byron screeched. "You only have one M-17!" His foot rose perilously close to Harry's half-constructed aircraft carrier.

Harry threw up a hand and shouted. "Don't you dare!"

I wrapped an arm around Byron's shoulders and pulled him back a step. "Would you stop, for cryin' out loud? The two of you! Why can't you be nice?"

"Mommy," Byron whipped around to face me, his full lip trembling with rage. He pointed at Harry and shook his finger as he enunciated each bitter word. "He's going to *kill my men!*"

Harry shrugged. "They have to die. They're enemy spies."

Byron uttered an inarticulate cry, something like *"orruggha,"* and lunged for Harry. Harry leaped up, his hands like blades, his right foot cocked in the air, poised to defend the ship.

Catching Byron in mid-leap, I tossed him on the big bed with a roar.

"*Damn-it!*" Then I made Harry return Byron's soccer men to their Lego field and join Byron on the big bed. They moved with alacrity. When I got into the *Damn-it* mode, they knew they were in trouble. Byron folded his arms and turned his face away with a *hrumph* and a frown.

"What's the matter with you two," I screamed. "Don't you realize that when Daddy and I are gone, all you are going to have is each other? When we're dead, you two will be all the family you've got!"

Now they were both frowning and blinking fast, and I realized immediately that this was not the appropriate thing for a parent to say. Nor would screaming at them that my only brother, their only uncle, was dying of addictive idiocy and they'd better appreciate having a brother while they've got one probably be the best way to help them toward brotherly love, either. But I had to find the words, the way to help them toward a place of love and health.

Grabbing each of them by the hand, I knelt on the bed, and – shaking their hands earnestly – I said, "Listen, I love each of you very, very much and each of you is made out of me and Daddy all mixed together and that makes you part of us, and it makes you a part of each other, too, and when you do things that hurt each other, you hurt me and you hurt Daddy and you hurt yourself. We're a family, and that means we love each other and we try to help each other and be good to each other."

Now the boys were looking down. Byron, having replaced his evil eye with a pout, muttered, "He was going to *kill* my men!"

Harry said, "I wasn't going to *kill* them; they were just going to be *injured*."

Definite progress. This was definite progress. From murder to mere wounding. I glanced at Harry gratefully. "Yeah, and maybe you guys could even play something without any war at all!"

But obviously I'd pushed beyond the pale. "No *war*?" Harry glanced up at me, aghast.

Despite my blunder, I could sense an overall loosening of tension. "See, Byron," I urged, "Harry wasn't really going to kill your guys."

"Yeah," Harry said to Byron, leaning around me enthusiastically, "and don't you have that new medic guy? That new GI Joe medic?"

"Oh, yeah," Byron beamed immediately. "My new medic!"

"You could heal them after the grenade goes off."

Both beaming now, they scrambled off the bed to retrieve the new medic GI Joe doll. "Get a bunch of grenades," I heard Byron shout excitedly. "Let's blow 'em sky high!"

"Get the Red Cross ship," shouted Harry.

There was a piercing whine of a falling bomb, followed by a growling explosion.

Byron came back in to pat my hand. "Don't worry, Mommy," he said. "It's just pretend."

"Uh-huh," I said.

"You know," he said, "since we all evolved from the earth, and since we are all a part of God, we are really *all* one big family, you know."

"Uh-huh," I said.

"That's why people really shouldn't have war," he said. "But don't worry. Harry and I are just playing. We know it isn't real."

There was a little tickle at the back of my throat and I didn't know whether I was going to cough or laugh or sneeze or cry. Instead, I went into Sean's music room, took off his ear phones, and kissed his ears, which earned me a hug and a smooch on the back of the neck. I listened to him play old Beatles tunes. *Love is all there is.* It was two hours past bedtime when we all finally went to sleep. Nobody did the dishes.

TEN: DOWN TO THE BONE, 1971 – 1979

*B*EHIND me, the stairwell door closes gently. I slide down the edge of the steps like a wraith. There is a sound below. I freeze. The sound of coins dropping. The echo of a soft thud. Footsteps. Silence.

Then I am alone under the burning blue lights. I feed the college dormitory machine my quarters, pull the magic levers, slip cupcakes and cookies into a plastic bag. Back in my dorm room, I eat them all, enough to make me sick. I can't stop. In six months, I gain twenty-five pounds. Food rots in my stomach; poisonous belches erupt from my gut, stinking. I try to throw up, but can't. Nobody knows, not even my boyfriend. I grab the fat around my middle and rend it, hitting and pulling as if I might rip it off. I fall onto the bed and scream my self-hatred into my pillow. How could this happen to me? I starve myself, then binge again. I watch another girl from my college dorm blow up like a balloon, then suddenly melt like hot butter down to the bone, then get fat all over again. I know it's a sickness.

The cycle of bingeing and starving myself does not end until I ask for help. My boyfriend and my therapist at college help me go on a reasonable diet. After a year, the mad cycle of bingeing and starving finally subsides.

Another student, an overweight girl with dark black hair and hooded eyes, doesn't make it. She works in the college coffee shop, and sometimes I see her eating on the side, a hastily gulped piece of pie. Other times, I see her sketching with charcoal; she can draw anything. I have been told that she has diabetes. Late one afternoon, I see her eating ice cream in the basement of the dorm. She turns away from me and walks the other way. She dies the year after we graduate.

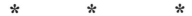

Some people are the first ones in their families to go to college. I am the first one in my family to go to therapy.

Slowly, over the years, I begin to recover. I dream I am in the devil's office, lying down on a hard couch. The devil is sitting beside me in an armchair. I am sobbing into my hands, my whole body squeezed and wrung with grief.

"I feel like I am such a bad person," I say to the devil.

The devil holds a pad of paper and a pencil in his hands. He is scanning the paper. "You're not on my list," he says.

I continue to sob. "But I feel like I'm such a bad person."

"No," says the devil, shaking his head, checking his list again. "You're not on my list at all."

I leave the devil's office and go out into the anteroom, a small, plain room without windows or adornment, where I pause as this news sinks in. I am not on the devil's list! A light without source fills the room and bathes me with unutterable joy.

*   *   *

Carter still idolizes our father, but that's because Carter lives in California. What does he know about the truth? What does he know about what happened to me! He doesn't even understand what happened to him.

One day, unexpectedly, I become free. It is the day I find my growl. It is my twenty-seventh birthday, and Caroline, my niece Emma, my friend Annie, and I are at Mom and Dad's house to celebrate. Carter is still in California, but he calls to wish me happy birthday. He wishes he were here, and I wish I weren't. I'm starting to feel depressed.

Outside the window, in the five o'clock dusk, on the small patch of blue-gray snow next to the spruce and the fir, my sister Caroline and Emma, who is eleven years old now, are making Swedish snow caves. I assume they're Swedish, anyway, because Caroline and Emma learned how to make them when they lived in Sweden years ago, before Caroline's divorce.

Each cave is made of snowballs that are built up into a small igloo. Inside is a candle, and as the night comes, the candles are lit. The light flickers and glows warmly through the chinks in the snow cave.

Later, as we sit near the windows to eat dinner, a melancholy takes me. The lovely snow caves glow red and yellow, and remind me of children. I feel the clock ticking. I long for a family of my own. But there is still plenty of time. Isn't there?

Dad is drunker than a skunk. He is behaving like a perfect ass.

"Wheee," he says, throwing shreds of his napkin up across the table. He disappears for five or ten minutes, then returns, reeking of vodka. There is no alcohol on the table, as usual. We never drink at home. Our whole family pretends that we don't drink.

"Hey," says Dad. "Let's go out … play out in the … schnow."

It is unusual for him to slur his words. He must be extraordinarily snockered.

We all look out the windows into the chill February night. It looks very cold.

"Nah, I don't feel like it," I say.

My father stands up, wavering, his nasty, drunken eyes narrowing at me. "Well, you're a fuckin' downer!"

Something in me snaps. It is something that has never snapped before and when it does, I am suddenly in a brand new place. I stand up, my own eyes blazing. "You're drunk!" I spit the words at him.

My father, lurching, leaves the room without a word, knocking silverware from the table as he goes.

It is amazing. It is the first time in my life I have ever confronted my father. I can't believe how easy it was. And the funny thing is, I don't feel bad at all. In fact, I feel really good.

I turn to the others at the table. "I'm sorry to ruin the party, but I just can't let him talk to me like that any more."

The others at the table put up their hands and shake their heads. "It's okay. Really. Don't worry about it." They don't mind.

"It is my birthday, after all."

Yes, everyone agrees. It is my birthday, after all.

ELEVEN: TOOLS OF RECOVERY
March

*B*YRON was running a fever and got to stay home. Harry complained bitterly about how healthy he was. "I'm not going to eat healthy food any more," he stormed. "I'm too healthy. I never get sick. Is he going to watch television?"

Harry glared at Byron, who had an unfortunate little smile playing around his lips.

"Byron is hardly ever sick," I soothed Harry, moving in front of Byron to block the view. "Remember you got sick just after New Year's? You stayed home then. Byron hasn't been sick all year."

Harry fumed all the way into the kitchen. "I'm not going to eat healthy food any more. All the other kids eat junk food. *Everybody* brings sweets for snack. Why can't I even have a Fruit Rollup? Nobody else in the whole school brings *an apple* for snack!"

Healthy food was a battle I had been waging against the public school system since Harry began kindergarten. My battle was motivated not only by Carter's food problems, as well as my own food problems, but also by the genetic health-bomb in our family. I could at least have some control over my children's *food*, couldn't I?

The 1990s saw a lot of federal bruhaha over revising the food pyramid and improving school lunch, but I don't think it trickled down to the local level. For example, somehow our school officials had the notion that it was necessary to have dessert after every meal. That is, if the meal itself was not dessert. Breakfast, for example, in the school cafeteria was usually a dessert meal: either sugar-coated cereal or some bready stuff in a pool of syrup. Lunch was pizza (tomato sauce is a vegetable, isn't it?) and ice cream. With chocolate milk. Or fried chicken nuggets with sugar-saturated corn and overcooked green beans, cookies, and ice cream. With chocolate milk.

Then there was that requisite, extra elementary-school meal every morning. It was called "snack."

In our neighborhood, snacks sent from home were Twinkies, cupcakes, or cookies. Moms who were especially health-minded baked their own cookies. Another "healthy" snack, I was informed by my children, was Fruit Roll-ups. (Which, according to the package, were made of corn syrup (a form of sugar), dried corn syrup (another form of sugar), sugar (yet another form of sugar), and pear concentrate – a very sugary fruit.) Accompanying snack were various juice packs that guaranteed they do, actually, amidst the corn syrup and water, contain some juice.

One time, when Harry was in kindergarten, in a moment of weakness I bought him a package of chocolate-chip trail mix at the deli. His teacher said he was so excited at snack time that he burst the package open in a frenzy, and the trail mix spilled all over the floor. O, the bitterness of tears when the chocolate chips are in the garbage! It was an early-childhood trauma he never forgot. After that, I stuck to the self-packaged, albeit despised, fruit. "Fruit has sugar in it," I told the children. "It's called 'fructose.' "

"That's not *real* sugar," the children whined hysterically. "Everybody else gets *real* sugar."

Instead of zero-tolerance for violence at school, I wished they had a zero-tolerance for sugar. No sugar allowed within 100 yards of school property. Five days' detention for anybody walking onto school grounds with brownies in her backpack. What was it with school lunch? In my day, there was no school cafeteria at all. If they were trying to provide healthy food for disadvantaged children, what the heck did they need sugar for? Over a period of four years, I watch with horror as the beautiful, sweet faces of my children's kindergarten classmates blew up into bulging balloons. Big fat cheeks. Big fat tummies. Big ballooning behinds. T-shirts too tight around the arms. Sweat pants binding over the thighs.

Don't these people see the smoking gun? By fourth grade, I estimated one third of the children from Harry's kindergarten class were obese. That was seven children out of twenty-one. Another third were beefy – "well-fed" as they say. Like cattle. Here I saw heart disease in the making. There I saw diabetes. Pulmonary disorders, joint disorders, gall-bladder removals, difficult pregnancies, kidney trouble, maybe a little cancer thrown in. Not to mention teasing and low self-esteem. Although I wondered if children were still teased for being heavy, since fat seemed to be the new norm.

"I'm too skinny," raged Harry. "My throat is sore. Don't let Byron watch TV!"

I lured him out to school with two bright quarters for ice cream after lunch. His consolation prize and hedge against being too healthy.

As soon as Byron was set with his water, his Tylenol, his crackers and peanut butter, his Gatorade, and his GI Joe, as the strains of *Star Wars: The Empire Strikes Back* began to recede behind the kitchen door, I got a spate of call-backs, in rapid succession, from the rest of Carter's doctors and nurses.

The first one to call was Carter's GP, Dr. Wave. He had a deep masculine voice with a nasally but well-articulated drawl. He sounded wealthy and exceedingly relaxed. My hackles rose as soon as I heard his voice. "Yes, hmmmm," pondered Doctor Wave, "well, nooo doubt, it would help his overall condition if he did loooose some weight." The way he drawled out the "no" in the "no doubt" and the "lose" in the "lose weight," you would think the preponderance of emphasis itself might help Carter shed pounds.

"What I'm hoping to find is some kind of a rehabilitation center, you know, like they have for alcoholics who want to quit drinking. Some kind of a rehab for obesity."

"Mmmm," proclaimed Doctor Wave. "Good idea."

"Do you know of one?"

"Noooo."

"What about gastric surgery. Do you think gastric surgery might help Carter?" I picture Carter's stomach stitched up like a red velvet pocketbook, the greater portion of it collapsed floating forgotten in the darkness and only a bright piece smaller than my fist still making change on a daily basis.

"I do know a few who had the suuurgery," said Doctor Wave, "and they are very uncomfortable, very sooooorry they did it at all." Doctor Wave was shooting down all my ideas and not offering a smidgeon of help and I was just about to get really annoyed with Doctor Wave and say something very rude, when it suddenly occurred to me that he was not affecting an upper class, Boston Brahmin drawl. His voice caught on his words the way a hanger caught inside a loose garment just as it is about to slide out, then doesn't. Doctor Wave, I realized, was fighting a stutter. He hung onto his words until they came clean. "Oh," I said in a small voice, blushing on my side of the receiver, glad I had not been nasty. "Thank you so much for your advice."

"Sooorry I couldn't be more help," he said. "Call me aaany time."

I decided Dr. Wave was nice a nice person after all, and I was *very* grateful I had not been rude. It just goes to show, I thought. You should never be nasty to anybody until you know them really well.

Dr. Remmy, Carter's cardiac surgeon, talked very fast in a high-pitched voice. I pictured him looking like a rabbit with black hair and glasses. "No, no," he said, "gastric surgery is not a good option for your brother. His overall condition is much too fragile for gastric surgery."

"Well, do you know of any detox or rehab for obesity?"

"No, I've never heard of a detox for obesity. He doesn't need a detox. He just needs to stay on his diet. If he stays on his diet, he will lose the weight."

I could see Doctor Remmy Rabbit twitching his chilly nose and adjusting his glasses. Easy for him to say, just stay on your diet. I'll bet dollars to dimes Doctor Remmy had never had a weight problem. Doctor Remmy Rabbit had no other words of wisdom, and his call was closely followed by Carter's other cardiac surgeon, Doctor Hillsenblatt.

Doctor Hillsenblatt had a gruff, booming voice, the voice of boundless energy and bright green vegetables. "Surgery's the thing!" said Doctor Hillsenblatt. "Gastric surgery. Amazing results. I've never heard of any kind of detox or rehabilitation center for obesity, but those kinds of things just don't work, anyway. The gastric bypass is having great success."

"But what about his heart?" I asked.

"Perhaps he could have bypass surgery," suggested Dr. Hillsenblatt.

"Another bypass?" I asked. "Uh, you know Carter had quadruple bypass surgery ten years ago?"

"Ah," said Dr. Hillsenblatt, "Well, then. Perhaps angioplasty. Or maybe some stents would help."

As I paused, groping for the appropriate words to express my dissatisfaction with his cavalier attitude, Dr. Hillsenblatt took my silence to mean the conversation was over and he hung up.

Next call back was from Eleanor Hodges, the nurse from Boston Memorial Hospital & Rehabilitation Center. Eleanor had a very sympathetic and sorrowful voice filled with Bostonian inflections that cracked her vowels open to all sorts of abuse in the back of her throat. In my mind, she looked like the kindly Nurse Jane Fuzzy-Wuzzy who took care of Uncle Wiggly's rheumatic foot.

"I am so sorry to hear about your brother, dear. We only have a detox for substance abuse."

"No food abuse?"

"No, nothing for food now."

"I heard you had an obesity addictions program there. Isn't food a substance?"

"Well, I guess it is, but we don't have anything to help you out. In fact, we did have a detox here for obesity, but it was discontinued years ago."

"Do you know of any kind of rehab for obesity – anywhere?"

"I'm afraid I don't."

"Was it an insurance thing? The obesity program closing?" I asked.

"Maybe," said Nurse Eleanor Fuzzy-Wuzzy sadly. "I don't know. It was a great program. My own sister was here once!"

"Did it work for her?"

"Oh, yes," said the nurse. "But she died many years ago."

The book on Boston Memorial closed with a thud.

I could tell that the social worker from the Wellness Center in Israel Schlomberg Memorial Hospital was a very intelligent person as soon as she responded to my description of Carter. "Your brother sounds so creative," said Ms. Erika Parker. "All that talent and creativity going to waste! What a great sister you are to try and help him out."

"Well," I said modestly, "you know."

The Israel Schlomberg Memorial Hospital Wellness Center had a very special weight-loss program. It was a liquid diet, a unique formula that their doctors had created. "This might be good for your brother," said Ms. Parker. "He can lose a big chunk of weight really fast, and then continue with a conventional diet. That really helps with motivation, you know? Once the patients get a big chunk of weight off, they are really encouraged to stick to their food plan. With your brother's medical condition, though, I'm sure he will need to be seen every day while he's on the liquid diet."

"That's okay," I said excitedly. The hospital was only about ten minutes from where Carter lived in Bentham.

The more I thought about this diet, the more excited I got. I thought I might have found The Answer for Carter. I had found The Plan. Carter would go on this liquid diet *for the rest of his life*. Carter would *totally give up eating.* Never eat again. He would do this liquid diet and then he would juice other foods. Even meat! I would give him Sean's juicer, another small appliance that needs constant cleaning with which I would be happy to part. And Carter would go to OA meetings to help him stick to the plan.

I was burning to put this plan into action. Now that I had the hospital and the diet, the next step was OA. I had to figure out this problem with OA and the "gray sheet" meetings so I could get Carter to go back to OA.

This OA "gray sheet" diet was a bunch of hooey, and I knew it. You should be able to do any diet at OA. Overeaters Anonymous was listed in the local phone directory, and I called to ask somebody. There was a warm and pleasant message on the answering machine, encouraging me to leave my name and number. Just as I begin to do so, a man named James picked up the phone. James had a lovely, deep, resonant voice. I pictured him tall, dark, and handsome. Definitely not overweight.

"Oh, we don't do gray sheet meetings around here," laughed James after I explained the problem. My heart leaped, triumphant. "Those guys are Nazis. They're very strict. We're very supportive around here. I'm sure they must have regular OA meetings around the Boston area where your brother is. Gray sheet meetings aren't really even regular OA. I'm sure there must be regular OA meetings your brother can attend."

I blubbered my thanks and suddenly resolved to go to an OA meeting myself. It was more likely that I could get Carter to go if I had my own experience to talk about. And after all, I had my own eating issues. James told me where to find an OA meeting that very night."You can't save him, you know," James said before we hung up.

"I know," I said defensively.

"I don't want to be harsh, but you can't save your brother if he doesn't want to be saved."

Oh yeah? I thought. *Oh, yeah?*

"Yeah, I know," I said aloud. "I think he wants the help."

"Well, if he wants the help, he'll take it. Otherwise, he'll find a thousand ways to avoid it."

"I know," I said, my mind already soaring with possibilities.

It was as I suspected! These gray sheet meetings were not legitimate OA. I jumped onto the Internet and pulled up OA's web site. Under "Tools of Recovery," the web site said:

> *There are no specific requirements for a plan of eating; OA does not endorse, recommend or distribute any specific food plan, nor does it exclude the personal use of one. For specific dietary or nutritional guidance, OA suggests consulting a qualified health care professional, such as a physician or dietitian.*

Ha, I said to myself. Ha! Gotcha!

There was a weird noise from the other room, and I suddenly remembered Byron. I ran into his room, but he was asleep in front of TV fuzz, all of the covers kicked to the floor. He must have cried out from a bad dream, but he seemed to be sleeping peacefully now. His head was still pretty hot, but it wasn't not too bad, about 101 F. This was one of my main talents as a mother, which I had honed to a razor-edged skill: I could tell my child's temperature to within half a degree just by feeling his forehead. It was lunch time, but I didn't want to wake him, so I turned off the TV, covered Byron up again, and raced back to the kitchen, my mind full of liquid.

Now I needed to find OA meetings for Carter to attend so that he could give up food and go on a liquid diet. It turned out to be easy. From information, I got the number of OA in Boston and they gave me a number for a contact in Bentham. I spoke to a really nice woman in Bentham who told me that there are many non-gray-sheet OA meetings around the area that Carter might attend. And, in fact, she gave me the times and places for five of them.

The excitement mounted as I felt myself closing in on a solution for Carter. Of course, I still had to talk to Carter about my solution. I had to convince him to give up food forever and go to OA meetings, but I was counting on the intervention to accomplish that. And, I was thinking, since there wasn't any rehab that Carter could go to, maybe I could actually go *and stay with Carter* to get him started. I could help Lyndsey out and take Carter to meetings and keep him occupied so he didn't eat. The plan solidified in my imagination: I would convince Carter to quit eating forever and go to OA. The kids and I would live with Carter and Lyndsey for a while to help Carter get started. I would put the kids in school in Bentham, stay there Tuesday through Friday, then we'd go home on the weekends to see Sean and do the B&B. Then we'd go to New York City so I could teach on Monday night, then we'd go back to Bentham on Monday night after I taught so the boys could go to school on Tuesday.

To some, this might have seemed like an unrealistic plan. Even a preposterous plan. Certainly an exhausting plan. But to someone in my family, it would seem like a perfectly normal plan. Only a matter of timing, really. Timing and organization and making phone calls. And lots and lots of coffee. And I might have put this plan into effect if only I had not run into a small but significant snag.

Just I was getting the phone number for the Bentham public school system from long-distance information, something occured to me. Something about "Bentham." Something was wrong about "Bentham."

Sweat broke out on my brow and my throat went dry. Bentham. Was that the name of the place where my brother lived?

Carter had moved from Watertown, just outside Boston, only a few years ago, and I had been to his new house only a few times. Wasn't the town where he lived more like "Bettam"? Somehow it seemed to me that "Bentham" might be a little off.

Bentham?

Bettam?

With a feeling of dread, I looked at my address book. Carter did not live in Bentham. Carter lived in Bettam. I looked on my Massachusetts map. Bentham was about 30 minutes north of Boston. Bettam was about 45 minutes south of Boston. Bentham and the Wellness Center and the wonderful social worker and the amazing liquid diet were all a two-hour-and-thirty-minutes-round-trip drive away, a drive my brother could not make on a daily basis. I sensed liquid flushing down the toilet.

My God, these irascible New Englanders! So parsimonious, they couldn't even spare a few extra consonants to make their towns distinguishable! Bentham and Bettam? Who ever heard of names so redundant? What did they name their kids, Martha and Marta? Herbert and Hubert? Everything was a "ham" around there. Couldn't they throw in a couple of "bergs" and a "ville" or two?

Geography had never been my strong suit. In polite terms, you might say that I am spatially challenged. You could rearrange the furniture in my living room and I'd have to trip over it to realize something was different. Names were not really my forte, either. Nor was I great with dates. I have a hard enough time keeping up with the here and now, and I have to know all about the there and the before, too?

This entire ridiculous mistake began with my call to the Israel Schlomberg Memorial Hospital Wellness Center. The hospital (in Bentham) even had the same *area code* as Bettam! Two towns stretched across opposite poles of Boston: A New Yorker couldn't imagine it. Where the heck were all the people in Massachusetts? I imagine the population density of a trout stream.

I called back the liquid diet social worker at the Wellness Center again, Ms. Erika Parker.

"Hello," I said. "I'm the one with the brother?"

She remembered me immediately.

"I'm not sure my brother could get in there every day. Would he have to go to the clinic every single day?"

"Well," she said, "he does have to come in every day, but maybe he could do the liquid diet just for a few weeks."

"Actually," I said, explaining my idea of total abstinence as a way of dealing with food-addiction, "I was wondering if a person could do a liquid diet forever – you know, never go back onto solid food."

"Oh, no," she said, "over a longer period of time, a person wouldn't get all the nutrients they need on a 100% liquid diet. Besides, people get to a point where they just can't stand the liquid diet any more. I've seen people, when they finally get off the liquid diet and go back on regular food, they just go crazy. They start eating and they can't stop. That's why we often do a combination of the liquid diet and food."

"Oh," I said, feeling discouraged. I could picture Carter going crazy after a couple of weeks on the liquid diet a lot more clearly than I could picture Carter staying on a liquid diet for the rest of his life. Plus there was no way that, in his current physical condition, he could drive a few hours every day back and forth to a clinic. I was beginning to suspect that the liquid diet at the Wellness Center was not really The Answer for Carter. The social worker wished me a heartfelt good luck before I hung up. Good luck! *Bon chance.* Was there a chance? Had Carter got any luck left?

Of course, all of the Massachusetts OA meetings that I had lined up were out of the question now. They were all too far away from Carter's house. I was gearing up to call OA all over again, in Bettam this time, when I heard a noise from the children's room. Uh-oh, I thought, my eyes darting to the clock. *I had totally missed lunch!* The noise came again. A weird noise. Something like a hyena crossed with a cat. My hackles rose.

Byron was on all fours on the edge of the bed, his too-small Pokemon zipup pajamas straining at the shoulders, staring over the side with stark wide eyes, swiping at the air like an angry lion cub.

"Uhhhuhu!" Byron whined fearfully.

"What's the matter? What is it?" I rushed to the bedside and knelt, trying to get into his line of vision. "What is it, Byron? What's there?"

He rolled back onto the bed and rose to his knees, searching the ferocious air. His hands, hooked like a claws, swiped around his head. "Uhhhhuh," he screamed. "Uhhhhuh."

"Byron," I called. "It's just a dream, Byron. There's nothing." I held his hands, ran my hands over his cheeks, his arms. "There's nothing, Byron. You're dreaming. Mommy's here. I'm right here."

He looked right at me with blank incomprehension, ducked under my arm and slid off the bed. Then he was off. Little bare feet pounding the floor. *"Mommieeee,"* he wailed.

"Shit," I muttered, running after him.

He'd never had night terrors in the middle of the day before. In fact, he hadn't had night terrors in months. I figured it was because of the fever. "It's the fever," I said out loud to myself, because what I was really feeling was: *I'm a bad, bad mommy!* Why did my little boy have such terrible fears? Was it my bad mommy skills? Was it my bad family genes? Was it because I forgot to give him lunch?

He was in the living room. I tried to hold him, but he pushed me away and ran a few steps, then stopped and looked wildly around.

"What are you looking for Byron?"

"It's the …" he tried to say. "It's …" Then he was off again.

Was he awake or asleep? I had never really been able to figure it out. In some way, he was cognizant of where he was. He interacted with furniture normally, for example, running around tables, climbing up on the arms of the couch. He seemed to see me. Sometimes he would even try to speak to me. Yet he did not seem to sense the "me-ness" of me. Even as he saw me, he was still looking for me. And there were other things that he did see. Evil things. Things he must escape. Things that were invisible to the parental eye. Things a parent could only sense.

I filled a cup with water and chased after Byron again. He was back in the bedroom.

"Come on, get in bed," I soothed. I helped him to drink some water, stroking his head. He swallowed four big gulps, lay down, turned over, and went back to sleep. Later, when he wakes, he will not remember the dream. I will never know what possessed him. Never be able to slay the bad things that chased him. I'd do anything to fight his nightmares, but could I be wise enough to find them?

When he wakes up, blithe spirit, Byron will not even know he was sleepwalking again. I will give him lunch: chicken noodle soup, peanut butter and jelly sandwich, milk. He will eat two spoonfuls, a couple of bites, a sip. Eat, I will urge him as he slides back, wan but feverless, onto the pillows. Eat! It will make you strong!

"*Fruit Rollup*," he will mutter hoarsely from his deathbed, "*and a Yoohoo.*"

TWELVE: THIS MORTAL COIL, 1980 – 1986

*C*ARTER runs through girlfriends like a series of new and faulty vehicles. Some last a few months; others last a few years. Whatever his high school problem with girls was, it evidently has vanished. He once confided to me that, according to his girlfriends, he is a great lover, a bit of personal information of which I would rather not have been made cognizant. Whatever his secret, women just love Carter. He is never without female companionship.

He brings a brand new girlfriend to Mom's family reunion in St. Louis. I was hoping to meet Susan, the woman he'd been living with for three years in California, but I learn that they've broken up and he is already in love again. The new girlfriend, named Lynda, practices astrology for a living. Lynda greets Emma, Caroline's twelve-year-old, with hugs and kisses, as if they were related. Emma's arms hang back like awkward wings. My sister rolls her eyes at me.

I gaze down the long dinner table at my cousins, most of whom I barely know. They all live in the South. There are children of my mother's brother, who died of alcoholism. There are children of my mother's sister, who also died of alcoholism. They are children of my mother's cousin, who is married to an alcoholic. There's no escaping the family disease.

Dad is not drinking right now, and that is a wonderful relief. I have not seen him in a few months, and he is looking good. He tells me about winning an Emmy for daytime TV. "It's awful," he says. "Everybody hates you when you win." Poor Dad. He can't win for losing. He wants everyone to love him, and he doesn't know how to make it happen.

"Where's Carter?" I ask Lynda, who is sitting next to me.

"He's lying down."

"What's the matter with him?"

"He has chest pains after that hike we took, so he's lying down for a while." Lynda seems blasé.

"*Chest pains*?" I am horrified. "He has chest pains?"

"Only after he exerts himself."

"Jesus Christ, Lynda. That's angina. Chest pains after exertion is a symptom of angina. He's got to go to a doctor."

Lynda is taken aback. "A doctor?"

"Yes, that sounds like it might be a heart condition. If he has angina, he has to get treatment. I bet he still has high blood pressure. He has to lose weight and … I don't know, exactly. But he has to go to a doctor."

Lynda looks doubtful. "I don't think he'll go to a doctor."

"What do you mean, he won't go to a doctor?"

"Well, you know he doesn't believe in Western medicine."

I repress a snort. In my opinion, Western medicine is the best thing to happen to humanity since the invention of soap, but Carter has gone Native. Once he tried to cure my bronchitis with some foul smelling smoke that made me cough so bad I thought I'd break a rib. In fact, Carter is actually hostile toward Western medicine. It ignores an entire part of the person, says Carter. Western medicine has no soul.

"He meditates to make the pains go away," says Lynda.

"Try to make him see a doctor, Lynda," I tell her, feeling defeated already. "I'm sure it's angina. Make him at least see a doctor to find out." Maybe it isn't angina, I think. Maybe I'm making too much of it.

Down at the other end of the table, I see my father lift the glass of complimentary champagne, laughing. My heart sinks. That's the end of his sobriety.

Back in New York City, I brood and fret about Carter. Does he have a heart condition? Will Lynda make him go to a doctor? Why didn't I confront him at the family reunion? Finally, I write Carter a letter. I never hear anything back. Every so often, I worry about Carter. After all, what else can I do?

*   *   *

Perhaps Carter would not have gotten so sick if he had stayed to resolve his relationship with my parents instead of running away to the other side of the United States. I think the pain was too much for him. California glittered for him with the golden stars of love and community, but of course, wherever he went, there he was. Carter could not connect.

Carter ends up living in a tiny trailer in his ex-girlfriend Susan's driveway, out of work and out of ideas. He finally gives up, abandons California for good, and comes home to stay with our parents, deeply depressed.

When I go to visit one weekend, he barely speaks to me until I am about to leave to meet Annie and another girlfriend back in the city. We are going to a movie, and then I am going home. Although he has hardly said two words to me during the weekend, Carter wants me to stay. Suddenly, he is very angry. "You're selfish," he shouts. "All you think of is your self."

"What are you talking about?" I'm poised next to the couch, ready to take off. My mouth has gone dry and tinny. I am scared and I hate Carter and I wish I had never offered to visit. "It's just time for me to go home."

"You *always* had friends," he shouts, swinging around with his fists clenched. Carter knows nothing about me, I think bitterly, and he never has. He sees nothing beyond his own circle of pain. I am suddenly aware of how big he is. He could crush me with one hand. But he just storms out of the house to his car. Mom creeps into the living room. Dad isn't home, or Carter would never have made such a scene.

Carter is sitting in his car, which he has not turned on, with the door hanging open. It has started to snow again. Carter falls sideways on the seat and does not move.

"I can't take it, Ma," I tell her apologetically. "I've got to go."

"It's all right," says Mom. "Go ahead and do what you have to do."

"He's going to freeze out there."

"I'll get him to come in."

"I saw him standing at the front door last night, in the middle of the night," I tell her. "I woke up. I think he was crying."

Mom makes a noise, but she is looking away and I can't tell what it means.

"Listen. He is really depressed. I think you better take him to the hospital."

"He doesn't want to see a psychiatrist."

"It doesn't matter what he wants. He's sick, Mom. He needs some help."

Mom nods. "Okay."

"Take him to the hospital. Force him."

"Okay," she says.

I know she won't do it. I get in my car, and I don't look back.

*　　　*　　　*

Soon after our car-in-the-snow blow-out, Carter meets and moves in with Maria, a woman who lives near my parents. After he meets Maria, Carter is absolutely fine. He is in love, and all is right with the world. It is as if he were never depressed. He starts a small, one-man home-improvement business; he joins the local theater group. Nobody mentions his weight. Nobody mentions his depression. He is happy. Why rock the boat?

On the train to Carter and Maria's house, I write a card for my father's birthday. He has finally gotten sober in AA, and I want Dad to know how much it has meant to me. At Carter's sumptuous spaghetti dinner, Dad reads it aloud:

Birthday
There you put down the drink
and there you gently lay aside the old self-hate.
I put my hand into yours, because, at last,
it is open.
If you were a man drowning, now
you are rising to the surface of yourself ...

Dad bursts into tears, unable to continue reading.

In a blaze of candles, Carter sings, "Happy Birthday," bearing cake and gallons of ice cream.

*　　　*　　　*

There is a famous story in Alcoholics Anonymous. It goes like this: Living with an alcoholic is like living with an elephant in your living room. Everybody comes and goes and chats and lives in the house as if nothing weird were going on. But there's this huge, gigantic elephant in the living room that everybody has to walk around. We just pretend it isn't there. In fact, we never, *ever* mention the elephant in the living room – it would be so rude. Don't talk about it. Just walk around it. Even when it stinks!

That's how we used to treat my father, and that's how we treat Carter. Like an elephant in the dining room. We have family dinners and look away when he has third helpings. Even when it stinks.

*   *   *

It is after ten at night when I get the call. I fumble in the dark for the phone.

"I'm sorry if I woke you," says my mother.

My heart is pounding. "What's wrong?"

"It's Carter," she says. "He had a heart attack."

I jump out of bed. "I'm coming."

"No, don't. He's stable for now. They're transferring him tonight to New Haven."

Early in the morning, I go to the New Haven hospital by train. Carter takes my hand as I stand next to him, the oxygen tubes in his nose. "I don't want them to operate," he whispers hoarsely. His fingers are weak in mine.

"Carter, Western medicine is what's going to save you now. Surgery can help you."

As an alternative, the doctor offers him angioplasty – the little balloon to blow up his collapsed arteries. But they don't know how long angioplasty will last, or if it will be enough. All four of Carter's arteries are clogged, one for each of his four decades. "You'll be awake through the whole thing," says the doctor reassuringly.

"Can't I get anesthesia?"

"No, you have to be awake for angioplasty."

"Why?" says Carter.

The doctor explains the procedure.

"I want anesthesia," says Carter.

"Mr. Watson, as I explained, the procedure can't be done with anesthesia. You have to be awake so that you can help us position the instruments."

"Why can't you use sonogram technology to position the instruments?"

The doctor breaths hard. "We don't do it that way, Mr. Watson."

"Does it hurt?"

"As I said, you will feel some discomfort. That is how we tell when we are in the right spot." The surgeon smiles tightly and looks at his watch. "I'm sorry, I have other patients waiting."

"I can't deal with the pain."

"Many people go through this procedure, Mr. Watson. The pain is not unbearable. It's more like, a, discomfort."

Carter shakes his head. "I don't see why you can't use a sonogram. You use that to guide the needle for amniocentesis. Why can't you use that to guide the catheter for the angioplasty?"

"Mr. Watson, if you don't want the angioplasty, we need to schedule the surgery as soon as possible. As I said, I think surgery is a better option for you anyway,"

"I want to do the angioplasty. I just want you to use anesthesia."

In disgust, the doctor leaves to see his other patients. I walk with him into hallway. "Your brother has to make a decision," the doctor tells me. "If he wants the bypass, we need to schedule it right away."

"I think he's afraid," I say meekly.

"Ms. Watson, if your brother took that oxygen out of his nose and walked away, he would collapse after two steps," says the doctor. "He has to do something."

Back in the room, I say, "Carter, they will *not* give you anesthesia for angioplasty. It's just not going to happen."

"How much do you think I'll feel it?" Carter asks, looking scared.

"I don't know, Carter. The doctor said it would hurt. Maybe it won't be too bad."

"Tell them to schedule the bypass," he says, letting go of my hand. He turns his head away, defeated. "I want to sleep through it."

They perform quadruple bypass surgery, using the mammary artery and a vein from his thigh to go around the blocked arteries.

In the elevator, going down to the cafeteria, my father bangs his head against the metal wall. "Why? Why? Why?"

People in the elevator stare at him.

"Jack," my mother says dryly, "we're *all* suffering."

I edge away and pretend I belong to another family.

*   *   *

Slowly, Carter recovers from his heart attack and bypass surgery at my parents' house. I take him into town for lunch.

"Let's go to that vegetarian place," I suggest.

"Oh, no, that stuff's awful tasting," says Carter. "Let's get pizza."

My insides freeze. "Carter, don't you have to ... you know ... change the way you eat?"

"What does it matter!" Carter says bitterly. He has fallen into another depression. He has broken off his relationship with Maria, and now he seems again lost and disconnected.

"Look, the doctor said you would even be able to ski again," I argue. "But you've got to, you know, get healthy. Lose some weight."

"I quit smoking!"

"Well, this vegetarian place has some kind of pizza. Why don't we try that?"

Carter makes a face and refuses. We compromise on hamburgers, and I go home in a funk.

It's hopeless, I think.

*   *   *

My father sits with Carter at the kitchen table. He is trying to stumble through something new, something he has learned in sobriety. "I'm sorry, Carter, uh, about, uh, everything."

Carter shakes his head. "About what?"

"Just this ... heart ... surgery and all ..." My father's voice starts to tremble.

"Pa ..."

"And I wish ..."

"It's all right, Pa."

"Well," says my father, wiping his eyes. "You wanna go on this diet together?"

"Okay," says Carter.

*   *   *

Carter loses forty-five pounds and starts taking antidepressant medication. By the following winter, he can ski again. Though he is still heavy, he is fluid and graceful on skis. When we ski together, I realize that Carter is a great teacher. He is awful at listening to other people, but he is great when he is in charge: encouraging, gentle, and articulate. At the top of Killington, amongst the fir trees, he corrects my stance and shows me how to turn. After twenty years as a beginner, I can finally brave the blue ice. Carter tells me he is going back to graduate school. He's moving to Boston to study Expressive Arts Therapy. He is going to be an Expressive Arts Therapist. He says he has finally found his niche.

THIRTEEN: BEAST IN THE COOKIE JAR
March

I was scouting Overeaters Anonymous for Carter. The OA meeting convened in the basement of the Temple Emmanuel. I waited in my car in the dark in the deserted parking lot, motor running, lights off. I didn't want anybody to see me trying to get saved. I used a penlight to read while I waited.

I'd begun a great book about recovery from food addiction that I discovered on Amazon-dot-com called *Holy Hunger* by Margaret Bullitt-Jonas. It was amazing how many things the author and I had in common. She binged, I binged. She wasn't really fat, and I wasn't really fat. She had an alcoholic father, and so did I. This book pulled no punches. She clearly identified her eating disorder as an addictive problem – something the medical establishment seemed to shy away from.

The really exciting thing about the book was that this woman had recovered from her addiction to compulsive overeating through Overeaters Anonymous. That meant the program really worked. I felt inspired to join OA for myself as well as for Carter.

But I was getting nervous. It was three minutes to seven. The meeting was supposed to start at seven and I had a bad feeling this meeting no longer existed. Too anxious to read, I waited in the dark, counting the minutes like calories, squeezing the paper bag from which I had withdrawn my supersaccharined decaf coffee with extra half-and-half. I pondered my earlier decision to *not* buy a Haagen-Dazs ice cream bar, which I easily could have finished by now in the quiet secrecy of my car. Now I was sorry that I hadn't, but later I would be glad. I thought about leaving the parking lot and driving back to the deli for the ice cream and coming back to the parking lot. But no, if the meeting really happened, I would not have time to eat the ice cream before going in. And, of course, I couldn't take an ice cream bar into my first OA meeting! Heaven forbid! I imagined a hundred pair of dark and hungry eyes riveted upon my mouth. Faces snarling like Bilbo Baggins as he glimpses The Ring hanging round Frodo's neck and the terrible lust rises, twisting Bilbo's sweet and trusted face into a mask of evil. *Urraguh! Gimme that Haagen Dazs!*

No, no, no ice cream at the OA meeting. I resolved my conflict with a promise to myself, actually a dodge, a stall: "We'll go and get the ice cream if the nasty OA people don't show up, won't we, my precious?" I said to the inner beast. "Nobody will know because they'll be thinking we're at the OA meeting."

"Yes, Yes," gruffed Gollum, all smarmy lip-licking and wringing its sticky hands.

But the beast was disappointed. At thirty seconds to seven, a car pulled into the black lot. Somebody got out and headed for the temple's basement door. I turned on my headlights and got out of my car. "Uh, hello," I called out. The woman turned around and pushed back a hood.

"Oh, hi!" she said. "Are you looking for the OA meeting?"

"Yeah."

"Right here," she said, proceeding to the door and unlocking it.

By the time I turned off my car, seven other vehicles had arrived and parked. I was swept into Temple Emmanuel's basement with the others. The people were chatting with one another, and I felt a little intimidated. I was not sure how to behave. What would happen next? Would they be mad at me when they found out that I was investigating OA for my brother? Should I pretend that I was there about my own food problem? Was I there about my own food problem?

It was cold in the temple, and the fluorescent lights shed a blue glare upon the room. We set up folding chairs. Everyone sat in a circle, and nobody even had coffee! I was *so* glad I finished mine in the car.

Once we were settled, I assessed the crowd. There were nine people, including me. One man and eight women. This worried me a little. Was OA mostly women? Would Carter feel comfortable in OA if it turned out to be mostly female?

Three of the people, including the man, were obese; five of us (including me) were middle-of-the-road; one was really skinny. The skinny one was wearing bulky clothes. You could tell she was skinny only from her face and her wrists, which had a lot of bones sticking out. I figured she was anorexic.

Questions raced through my mind. Were all of these people recovering from addictive eating patterns? Were they "abstinent" from compulsive overeating? How long had they been going to OA? Were the heavier people new, or was the program just not working for them?

Unfortunately, the answers remained a mystery. I hoped the meeting would begin with people talking about how they recovered from compulsive overeating, but the meeting began with reading from an OA book. When we are finished reading the chapter, everybody began to write in a notebook. This was a writing meeting. Somebody offered me some paper and a pen. What should I write about? I wrote about my brother and how I hoped OA will help him. It was quiet for some time – only the scratching of pens.

Then some people read aloud what they had written. One by one, the people at the meeting spoke or passed. When it came to me, I told everybody that this was my first OA meeting. Everyone broke into smiles and welcomed me. *Try several different meetings,* I was told. *Every meeting is different. Try several meetings before you decide.* I read aloud what I had written about Carter. There were nods and concerned looks. I hastened to add that I had my own eating problem with sweets, too. *Keep coming back,* they said.

When it was the obese man's turn to speak, he passed. I was very disappointed. Somehow, I thought he might have the answer for me. The answer for Carter. But perhaps he had no answers yet.

Then the meeting was over. We stood up and said a few words, then dispersed in our puffy winter gear like dandelion fluff on a breeze. I felt very disappointed and isolated. Not an encouraging reaction to my first meeting, I think. And I, unlike Carter, really *liked* group activities. No wonder Carter didn't like OA. And yet, I knew OA could work. People had recovered in OA.

In the parking lot, one of the women from the meeting stopped me.

Though she announced her name in the meeting, I'd already forgotten it. She was short like me and had short, iron gray hair and a firm handshake. I like her right away.

"Hi, I'm Peg," she said with a grin.

I grinned back. "Hi, Peg."

"That's great that you're trying to help your brother," Peg said. Our breath clouded on the air under the temple's back door light and drifted into darkness.

"Thanks."

"How did you like the meeting?"

Uh... I think. Should I be honest? "Well, uh, I was a little surprised nobody said anything about food."

Peg nodded. "Every meeting is different. This is a writing meeting. You might want to try a beginners' meeting," she said. "That's where they talk about the tools of the program."

"I can't figure out how all this can help people stop compulsive overeating."

"There are all different kinds of meetings," she repeated. "Every kind of meeting can help you with something different. You have to try several before you make a decision." She gave me the time and address of a beginners' meeting.

If Carter had come to this meeting, he would have hated it. He would have done what he did after the "gray sheet" meetings. He would have backed off; all the forward momentum would have been lost.

Maybe I was being unfair, but I felt annoyed with OA. How many people have tried OA once and failed to return? How many people with compulsive overeating were out there who might have been helped? If this meeting was not good for a beginner, why was it recommended to me?

I tried to suspend judgment until I could get to a few other meetings. On my way home, I stopped at Denise's house to complain.

"Oh, I tried that meeting once," said Denise.

My mouth dropped into a small o. I never knew Denise had tried OA. It made sense, though. She'd been struggling with her weight for a long time. Denise was so pretty, after a while you just didn't notice her weight. ("It's dangerous," I've said to her in the past. "Look what's happening to my brother." "Yeah, I know," she'd said casually. "I've been taking blood pressure medication for years.")

"You tried that meeting?" I asked.

"Yeah, I thought it was terrible."

"Why?"

"Because. It seemed totally useless."

"Mmm," I murmured noncommittally.

"And I felt very uncomfortable there. Like an outsider."

I sighed. "How am I going to help my brother if OA doesn't work?"

"Maybe it just didn't work for me."

"It worked for the writer of this book I'm reading. It seemed to work great."

"Well, try some of the other meetings. That's what they say, isn't it? Try different meetings before you decide?"

"Did you do that?"

"No."

"Mmm," I said again.

When I got back home, there was a message on the machine from Mom. Carter was home from the hospital. I called him up right away, even though it was late. He answered on the first ring.

"How you doing?"

"Pretty good," he answered cheerfully, and then launched into a litany of complications caused by his medications. The doctors seemed to have identified the imbalance that was causing his most recent problem and he was feeling much better now. The only thing that bothered me was that he sounded like he was out of breath. "I'm sorry I didn't get the diet to you," he said. "I was actually working on it right now." *(Puff.)* "I'm still trying to get the program installed." *(Puff, puff.)* "Then I've got to read through this whole book to figure out how to use it."

"Are you sure you're okay, Carter? You sound out of breath."

"Yeah, I'm fine," *(Puff, puff.)* "I just have to use the oxygen a little more."

I panicked. Was I even going to have time to get him to go to OA?

"Carter, guess what? I tried an OA meeting out here."

There was an ominous silence on the other end of the line. Not even a puff.

"Carter?"

"Mmm," he said, letting out a breath.

"So," I blundered forward. "It was good. There was no gray sheet or anything."

"No gray sheet?" Carter said, sounding surprised.

"No, no. Not at all. In fact, nobody does gray sheet around here. They all think the gray sheet people are a bunch of Nazis."

"Hm!" said Carter. "Around here, they're all gray sheet meetings." He sounded a little huffy, but I persisted.

"I'm sure there must be some regular OA meetings around there, Carter. From what I'm reading and hearing from other people, the gray sheet meeting is kind of a sub group. I'm not really even sure that it's legitimate OA." In my mind, I was setting up for Carter's new OA program. I would find him some good local meetings to go to, I would find him another man in OA that he could identify with, and I would launch him on a brand new OA path to recovery.

"Well, did it seem like any of the people at the meeting were really recovering?" challenged Carter.

"Well, yeah, I think so," I said, taken aback.

"Around here, if it's not a gray sheet meeting, the people are so accepting and relaxed and easygoing and everything, they don't have any recovery at all."

"Uh – really?"

"Yeah, they just go to meetings and don't lose weight."

"You mean you went to some non-gray sheet meetings?"

"Yeah. I went to one or two. They're useless. The people just sit around and talk about their problems and don't stay on a diet or lose any weight."

"Are you sure?" I was dismayed.

He must have heard the disappointment in my voice, because he modified his criticism at once. "Well, that's what it seems like around here, anyway. But maybe things are different over where you are."

"I know it's got to work in some places, because many people have been helped." I told him about the book I'd been reading about recovery from food-addiction. "In fact," I added, "the author comes from Boston. So there's got to be some recovery around there!"

"Well, could be," he said noncommittally.

"Anyway," I urged, "I can do any diet I want at OA around here. So whenever you get that diet program worked out for me, I'll be all set."

Now his enthusiasm returned. We again reviewed my vital statistics: age, height, weight, level of activity, goal weight. Carter was happiest arranging and fitting information together into orderly structures. In a way, it was a lot like my boys playing Legos. Locking the little random pieces together to create something substantial, something you can build on, something you can use. Why didn't Carter stick to engineering? He was seduced away by the lure of something infinitely more meaningful, but maybe he would have been happier if he had kept to the straight and narrow. It was good that he had ambition – too many young people today have none at all. But if only his ambitions had been a little less grand and a little more realistic. He kept trying to fit a new social order together like Legos, but it always fell apart.

Basically I blame Marcuse, Carter's favorite author at Cornell. All those overintellectualized idealists! Communism! It's hard enough to get a family to share. How are you going to force these humans to be good, I'd like to know? How're you going to make them share? How're you going to dictate love and respect? How are you going to eradicate individual desire and personal ambition? How are you going to get anything done if there *is* no individual desire and personal ambition? How many times has an idea looked like the ultimate grace on paper, only to create murderous totalitarianism in the flesh? I mean, are you telling me that you are going to create a community of human beings with no selfishness, no desire, no will to power, no urge to dominate? Either you give people the freedom to choose to be good or bad in their personal lives, or you create a monster for a government. Because the beastie part of human nature is going to pop out somewhere.

If only Carter had practiced the theory of dog-mind instead of reading Marcuse. If only he had been content to find his place in the pack. If only he had looked within, instead of looking in a book. If only he had been more honest with himself. He might at this very moment have been happily building bridges instead of constructing diets. He might have never gotten sick.

In a way, though, the ambition of Carter's vision was remarkable.

Since he was unable to fit into the pack, he decided to create a pack into which he could comfortably fit. Voila! A bright new sociological phenomenon. A sanctuary of love, peace and brotherhood within the competitive American capitalist empire. But when his community fell apart, Carter was alone.

This was why I felt I had to get Carter back into OA. It was his chance to rejoin the pack. His chance to redefine himself, to identify with others, to start anew.

"Carter," I said on an impulse. "I was thinking about coming up there to visit you for a couple of days. I mean just me, without the boys." I had this feeling if I could just get close to him, just radiate my love and good will, maybe it would make a difference. Besides, it would give me a chance to confer with Lyndsey about the local OA meetings, maybe even get Carter to try one out. "You can show me the whole diet then, you know. You can show me how it works."

"Uh," he hesitated, "what about the B&B?"

"Oh, you know, that's just weekends. There's nothing during the week."

Sean had wandered into the kitchen. He puckered his lips into an "o" shape, raised his eyebrows, and tilted his chin at the telephone receiver. This meant, "Who is it?" Sean, like many men I knew, communicated best with body language. Words tended to get muddled up with things like indefinite pronouns and choking sensations.

I covered the receiver with my hand. "Carter," I mouthed silently.

"The kids are in bed," he whispered to me proudly. This was a good thing, since it was 10:45 on a school night.

 "I'm going to go visit Carter, okay?"

Sean nodded vigorous approval.

Carter was still hemming and hawing. "I can't do very much, you know. I sleep a lot during the day."

"Yeah, I know," I urged. "I have a lot of work I can bring with me. I have to finish an article. I don't want to do anything anyway. It's just to visit you."

"Well, okay." He began to warm up to the idea. He was home alone all day long while Lyndsey was working, and I know that it had to be lonely for him. "That would be great, if you think you could get away."

"Great," I said. "How about tomorrow?"

"Tomorrow?" said Carter.

"Tomorrow?" said Sean at the same time, looking much less approving than he had a few moments ago.

"Yeah," I told Carter, looking pointedly at Sean. "This is the perfect time. Sean is laid off right now and he can watch the kids. I'll come tomorrow and go home the next day."

Sean nodded, his glazed eyes rolling back in his head as if gazing at a terrible vision of himself multitasking at 7 a.m. Something like trying to get the children to brush their teeth and put their shoes on at the same time you're trying to make school lunch and get the car warmed up. Sean shuddered.

Carter agreed. I would drive down there in the morning, spend the night, and drive back the next day.

"Make me a list," said Sean when I got off the phone.

"It's just getting them ready for school," I said, looking at the calendar. "Oh, and pick up Byron late, after his after-school program. Oh, but you better take his temperature in the morning. Don't send him to school if he's got a fever. Oh, and send a bag of nuts in with Harry. They're doing a special project. Oh, and make sure they do their homework. Oh, and …"

"Make me a list," said Sean.

I sat down on the bed and wrote a list as he gazed over my shoulder.

"How's Byron?" I asked. "He had another one of those sleepwalking things this afternoon. Some kind of terrible nightmare."

"He is much better," Sean proclaimed.

"Oh, is his fever down?"

"I don't know," said Sean, "but he was beating up on Harry pretty good when they were having a pillow fight."

As if on cue, Byron appeared in our bedroom. His hair was tousled and he was still wearing the too-small Pokemon pajamas. He entered the room squinting into the light, ran forward, and fell into my arms. "Mommy," he said, "I think I'm going mad."

"What do you mean?" I said, horrified. "What's the matter?" I felt his forehead. Normal. The fever was gone. "His fever is gone," I announced.

Byron clutched his hair. "I feel weird."

Sean crouched down. "What do you mean 'weird'?"

Byron looked around, spooked. "The silence sounds weird."

"He's having another dream," I said to Sean over Byron's head.

"No I'm not," Byron asserted aggressively. "I'm awake. See?" He opened his eyes very wide, pulling his mouth down and displaying his awake eyeballs, turning back and forth between me and Sean. "I haven't even been asleep yet. I can't go to sleep. I think I'm going mad."

"You're not going crazy," I said automatically, fear surging through my belly because the truth was, I was afraid that he *would* go crazy. "Why do you think you're going crazy?"

"The silence sounds weird."

"The silence sounds weird?"

"Yes," he said, clutching himself to me like a baby monkey.

"What does it sound like?" asked Sean.

"Weird," said Byron.

Sean and I looked at each other helplessly.

"He had one of those terrible dreams this afternoon," I offered. "It was very scary."

Sean stroked his head and scratched him behind the ears. "Don't be afraid. If you have a bad dream, you can come get in bed with us."

Byron turned around and looked at his father sternly. "I am not *afraid*," Byron admonished. "I am *concerned*!"

Sean and I nodded dumbly. "Oh," we said.

"Maybe he should get in bed with us now," I proposed.

Sean put some music on. "Listen to that, now," he said. "You won't hear the silence."

Between us, Byron fell asleep immediately to the muted strains of the latest Jeff Beck CD. After a while, Sean fell asleep, too. I turned the music off, but it was a long time before I could sleep. I lay there worrying about silence and sanity, trying to catch the pulse of the weirdness of the universe.

FOURTEEN: CHURCH OF MY SOUL, 1989 – 1993

I have just turned off the light when the phone rings. It is Mom. "Oh," she says, breathing hard.

"What's wrong?"

"Oh, I just can't believe it."

I turn the lights back on, filled with dread. "Just spit it out, Mom. Is somebody dead?"

"Yes," she says.

A terrible thought strikes me. "Emma?" She has again just gotten out of the hospital.

"No."

"Ma, who? Just say it. Spit it out."

"Poppie."

"Oh, no."

My father has dropped dead in the middle of an aerobics class at Canyon Ranch Resort in Tucson, Arizona, where he went to try to quit smoking. Massive heart attack.

Carter and I are devastated. Caroline is more ambivalent. She is still very angry with him. She can't believe he is dead. I can't believe it, either. Carter and I go to view the body when it is shipped back.

The funeral home is paneled with fake veneer. I have never been in one before. I have never seen a dead person before. You go through a vestibule and into a sitting room with stiff chairs. Toward the back there is another, larger room with long velvet curtains. At the back of the larger room is a coffin with my father lying in it.

I scream and my knees buckle as I catch sight of his waxen face. Carter catches me under my arms. I hide my face in my hands, turning away, terrified.

"You don't have to do this," says Carter.

"I can do it," I say. I wanted to see him. I needed to say goodbye.

Carter is crying, but I am crying out – a half scream, half sob, as if I were being cranked in a vise. The funeral home director hurries away from the terrible sound and stands outside the front door, smoking. The air rips out of my lungs, but Carter is not afraid of me. Carter holds me up, his arms under mine, and we move forward together until we stand in front of Dad.

As one, we kneel and weep. When we rise to leave, there is a new place in my heart that is forever Carter.

*   *   *

Three months later, I meet Sean. He grew up with an alcoholic father, too. By our second date, we are madly in love.

"Are we co-dependent?" asks Sean.

"Absolutely," I tell him.

"That's good," says Sean, tightening his arms around me. "You have to depend on somebody."

*   *   *

One year later, Carter visits Sean and me in New York City. He's come from Boston, where he is finishing graduate school in Expressive Arts Therapy. He has come to see his brand new nephew, Harry. I lie in bed and Carter sits in the chair opposite, the sunlight flooding in over his heavy, rounded shoulders. The tiny infant sleeps swallowed in his gentle arms. Carter croons, rocking.

After Harry was born, as I lay in the hospital for the second time in my life, a nurse said to me, "Now, you *will* get depressed." She smiled, like it was a promise.

I wondered if I should tell her I'd just spent the past fifteen years overcoming depression, or if I should just spit in her eye. What was it about me and nurses?

But of course, the nurse was wrong. How could she have possibly known? The devil himself told me I was not on his list. In my bedroom, the light floods through the window across my brother's shoulders, until the ceiling itself dissolves into a cascade of luminescence and fills my family – my brother, my child, and me – with unspeakable joy.

*   *   *

This church might be the one, thinks Carter. He likes the minister, and the service includes a lot of music. The church is not far from where he lives in Watertown, just outside Boston. He has tried several other churches that are further away. It would be good to join a church that is close to home.

He is thinking about this when the soloist begins to sing. She stands up and opens her mouth, and when she does that, he does not think any more. Instead, he is floating. Floating inside her voice. She is tall, her face striking and beautiful, but it is her voice that carries him away. This is the one, he knows. This woman is the one. The church of his soul.

After the service, Carter hurries to the vestibule to meet this amazing singer. He lingers until he can speak to her alone. Her name is Lyndsey. Carter grasps her hand, and they look into each other's eyes. Lyndsey feels something happen. The doors to her heart fly open. They are there together in this moment in time, and the worlds revolve around them, and click again into different spheres, a new universe where Carter and Lyndsey are one. Three weeks later, they become engaged. Six months later, they are married.

FIFTEEN: THE FINGER-WIGGLE EXERCISE PROGRAM
April

I pulled in behind Carter's car, a ten-year-old Jeep Wagoneer with a lift for the scooter attached to the back of it. The scooter itself sat next to the front steps covered in plastic, patient as an old dog. It looked like a geriatric motorcycle. It was plugged into an outdoor electrical plug, charging for the moment it might be needed.

Was I here to save Carter, or to say goodbye?

I walked from my car to the front door, the four flat strides that Mom and Caroline said Carter was barely able to make. I knocked, but not too loudly. He could be sleeping. We had arranged it ahead of time – if he were sleeping when I arrived, I would go to the back door and find the key. There was no answer, so after a while I walked down the steep hill to the back of his house.

The sun was just rising over the lake behind Carter's house. I could see my breath frost and drift toward the mist hovering over the dark water. I held perfectly still, hoping to see one of the blue herons that lived here. This was a beautiful place, but so isolated! Woods extended on either side of the house and rambled down to the water. There were other houses back there, but they were still hidden in small pockets of early morning darkness.

It was easy to find the key, barely concealed behind the picture of forget-me-nots that Carter painted in a fit of artistic enthusiasm. The painting was propped up against the back of the house, like something he kept meaning to throw away.

Inside the house, everything was shadowy. They were not expecting me so early. I picked my way through the lumps of darkness like an inveterate burglar, without a whisper of sound, and went up into the living room. There, I would stretch out under the warm, fuzzy throw and read my book, *Holy Hunger,* which I had decided to finish and leave strategically placed for Carter to discover.

The living room was a small square off the kitchen, with a daybed on the other side of the room from the couch, and a big armchair opposite the TV. The daybed was lumped up with shadowy blankets and clothes, so I stretched out on the couch, where to my delight I did find the fuzzy comforter, in which, evidently, my brother's dog Tripper had also been delighting. He growled for a moment, then licked my nose. I switched on the small reading light at one end of the couch and suddenly realized *I was not alone.*

Across the room, on the daybed, under a mound of blankets, a plastic nozzle clamped over his nose, I saw my brother, *and my brother's eyes were open wide, glassy, staring. Was he breathing? His chest was not rising and falling. In fact, he was not moving at all. He was dead.*

With a gasp, I leaped to my feet. Tripper also jumped up with a sharp bark. Carter sat up with a grunt and pulled the air hose off his face. "Hi," he said. "I didn't think you'd get here this early."

My heart was hammering away. He really had looked dead, and he still didn't look great. There were deep grooves from the air hose around his mouth, and his usually sparkling eyes seemed dull. He had a kind of looking-away look even when he was gazing right at me. He turned on the light by the daybed. His features seemed swollen and his skin was gray. He cleared his throat and ran his hands through his thinning hair. I wonder if it was a trick of the light. Could his skin actually be gray? His hair was definitely grayer than I remembered.

Since he hadn't been making the family holidays, and I'd been too busy to get away, I hadn't seen my brother in almost a year. The change was shocking. He had always been heavy, but Carter had always looked strong. Now he seemed weak. Weak and tired. His shape had lost all definition. He was not merely heavy; he was puffy. His eyes, his eyelids, his cheeks, his lips, even his ears. Everything was swollen. As he sat up, one thin spread fell from his shoulders, which were rounded and bowed inward by the weight of the world. The lumpy hillock I mistook in the dark for clothing or blankets was just him.

I tried not to show my dismay. Suddenly I understood my sister's urgency. There was not much time, I thought. I lowered my gaze, pressed my cheek to his, and though his cheek was warm, I had the feeling that there was a thick curtain of flesh hanging between my real brother and me. My arms embraced the citadel of his chest like trying to hold a tower, a massive castle that left me flung open wide, holding nothing.

We talked for a while of inconsequentials, the trip, the traffic, his dog's latest girlfriend. He told me he slept in here now, so that he wouldn't bother Lyndsey. He sleeps only a few hours at a time, then gets up for a few hours, then goes back to sleep.

Slowly, I got used to the new Carter. He smiled, he chuckled. The life came back into his eyes, the old spark. Not entirely gone, I saw. I could see him peering out from this other man's eyes, still in there.

When I was little, though Carter and I fought tirelessly, we did occasionally play together, and we always played the same game. It was Carter's game, in which he was a horse (or some other means of transportation) and I was a rider. Since he was so big and I was particularly tiny for my age, he made an admirable steed. Whether I was King Arthur riding into battle, or *Tom Corbet, Space Cadet* rocketing to save planets, or Mogli hunting Sher-Kahn atop an imposing elephant, Carter always played the supporting role in his own fantasies. As my powerful and trusty (not to mention exceedingly smart) horse (or rocketship or elephant), he'd keep up a running dialogue on what I was supposed to do next to defeat the enemy. Brave and wiry warrior that I was, I rose to the occasion and slew whatever ghostly foes presented themselves in our broad back yard.

Now could I slay the enemy that accosted him? And would he play a supporting role?

I yawned hugely. The conversation had turned back to Tripper, who at age eleven was a rather overweight snowball the size of a boulder who thought he was a lap dog. Carter was telling me about Tripper's diet and the vitamins and supplements Tripper ate now – something about elder-doggie kidneys and bladders that I really didn't want to know.

"Speaking of diets," I said blearily, yawning again, "did you finish mine yet?"

"No," said Carter, looking up with enthusiasm. "I need to know what kind of activity level you want me to use. I mean, like for me, I use 'sleeping' 18 hours a day, because I'm so inactive now." He chuckled. "That's as much sleep as the program will let you get. I wish I could sleep 18 hours! Then I use 'watching TV' the rest of the time. That's the second most inactive you can get. So I get my 24 hours with the least amount of energy expended, and the program calculates how many calories I can have, how many grams of fat, and so on, all based on my size and age and how much activity I get. So you need to decide whether you are going to exercise or not and then write up a chart for an average day, you know, an activity chart for an average day so I can see how long you spend at each activity for a 24-hour period."

"Carter," I said as it slowly dawned on me. "Have you begun the diet?"

"Oh, yeah," he said, nonchalant. "I started it a couple of weeks ago."

My jaw hung down. "A couple of weeks ago!" I said. "I thought you said you didn't have it all set up yet. You told me... Don't you remember, you told me you didn't have it set up yet?"

Suddenly, I was suspicious. Was he lying? Was he "stretching" the truth? What was going on here?

"Yeah, well, I basically know what the diet is. I didn't get the computer program all set up until last night, actually. Once you get it on the computer, you can work out a new food plan every day. I was just using my old food plans from Systems House. Now I've got it set up, I can have more, you know, variety. I already lost ten pounds!"

"Wow, that's great!" I said encouragingly, my mind scrambling like a cornered rat. Carter had started a diet about five hundred million times. The problem was staying on the diet. "I can quit drinking whenever I want," says the inveterate alcoholic. "I've done it a million times!" That's why I wanted to do the intervention. Carter needed a real program, a community of recovery. OA was the answer for him. But how could the family gang up and kick his butt into recovery if he were already dieting?

Suddenly I felt incredibly sleepy. I leaned back on the couch and yawned big again, and Tripper joined me with a soporific drool. "I'm sorry. I only slept an hour before I started out."

"Go on and lie down," said Carter. "I've got to do some work for my lawyer." Carter was in the process of suing the people at the addictions in-take clinic where he worked until a few years ago. They encouraged him to work part-time after he'd been in the hospital and never informed him that his health insurance was going to be discontinued (since he was working part-time), so that by the time he found out and continued his health insurance on his own, his heart condition was listed as a "pre-existing condition" and all the bills weren't covered for the first year. Honestly, you have to be a minor genius to file everything you are supposed to file for health insurance. Sean says they should forget health insurance altogether and create a new system whereby the government pays for all the hardware (the hospitals and clinics, the equipment, and the medicine) and the individual people pay for the software (the doctors and the nurses). We could bring back the system of free-enterprise: Doctors' prices would be influenced by the open market. Who knows, they might even start making house-calls again! Of course, you would have to allow the lawyers and the insurance executives to tear each other's hearts out, but hey, only their mothers would miss them, right?

I fell back on the couch and pulled the fuzzy comforter away from Tripper again, swooning into the circular argument whipping around my head: *If Carter got better on his own, then we didn't have to help him, but if we didn't help him, he might not really get better on his own, but if he were getting better already, wasn't it better to let him do it on his own, but if doing things alone was part of the problem, then wasn't it better to help him?* With Tripper's claws tucked up under my rib cage and his nose pressing against my kidneys, it took me about 30 seconds to pass out.

When I awoke, the house was quiet. Sunlight was flooding in. It was 11:30. Lyndsey had already left for work, and Carter was sleeping again on the daybed, the plastic oxygen-hose nozzle obscuring most of his face. I took advantage of this opportunity to strategically place the book *Holy Hunger* on the coffee table where Carter couldn't fail to see it when he woke. I also left some of the OA literature I got from the meeting strewn around as if I had been reading it. I called Sean at home and found out that Byron was okay and in school, no nightmares last night, and Sean hoped I would come home as early as possible tomorrow.

I was looking at the coffee table with all the OA literature and as soon as I got off the phone, I collected it all again because it was too obvious. Carter would know I was trying to get him to go to OA. Then I put it in a neat little pile next to the couch. Then I stuffed it all back into my suitcase again and only left out the *Twelve Steps of OA* book and the pamphlet, *Is OA Right for You?*

Diet or no diet, I had to get Carter into OA. He had to have some kind of life-changing experience to be able to stick to his diet. I would still go forward with some kind of a family intervention. We had to stop bullshitting. We had to tell him he's an addict who needs help. He just couldn't do it alone.

That night there was an OA meeting nearby, one that was not a gray sheet meeting, and I had decided that I was going to try to get Carter to go to it with me. In fact, this was one reason I wanted to be at his house on a Tuesday. I was hoping to get one of the people I'd spoken to on the telephone to show up at the meeting also, so Carter could make a friend, get connected. I was especially hoping the man I spoke to would come to this OA meeting. I made a few phone calls and left messages on answering machines. "We'll be at the meeting tonight," I murmured to the electronics. "It would be great if you could meet us there."

Then, with great care to be as quiet as possible, because the kitchen is not far from where Carter was sleeping, I began to check out the cabinets. The last time I was here, the kitchen was stocked with low-fat coffee cakes, low-fat cookies, candy bars for diabetics, low-fat individual mini-apple pies, low-fat ice cream, Weight Watchers ice cream sandwiches (I've tried those, they are pretty good if you eat three fast), different bottles of flavored pancake syrup made with ersatz sugar, low-fat pancake mix, and so on. I suppose if you ate any of these diet foods individually and in moderation, they would be better for you than eating the regular stuff, but Carter was just not a moderate kind of guy. Instead of helping his diet efforts, these foods – many of them high in calories and carbohydrates – just allowed him to pretend he was dieting when he was constantly overeating.

But as I checked, I found none of the regular fattening foods around, and none of the diet foods, either, except for diet soda. Just meat, vegetables, whole-grain bread, fresh fruit, skimmed milk. Frozen juice bars instead of ice cream. Well, several boxes of NutraSweet instant pudding, but it was very low calorie. Had Carter truly reformed? Gone on the wagon? I couldn't believe it. I snuck into the bedroom and looked under the bed, not realizing that Carter couldn't get down on his knees to hide stuff under the bed any more. Peeking into the living room and ascertaining that Carter was still asleep, I guiltily began to poke through more intimate stuff – drawers, closets, the medicine cabinet. Carter's house was small, and there were not many places to look for stray cupcakes. The whole place looked clean! The phone rang as I was poking around in the hamper in the bathroom (Carter does all the laundry), and I sprinted to pick it up after the first ring. It was Lyndsey.

"Hey," she said, explaining she didn't want to wake me before she went to work.

"Carter's asleep," I told her in hushed tones.

"Yeah, he usually is around this time. He doesn't sleep half the night. I just wanted to say hello." She sounded curious and I knew she was wondering what I had up my sleeve.

"Lyndsey," I said, hardly able to contain myself, "is Carter on a real *diet*?"

"Well, maybe. I think so," she said. She began to whisper also. "He said he was going back on that Systems House diet a few weeks ago, but he was cheating the whole time. And then we had a *big* talk."

"A big talk?" I urged excitedly. "When? What happened?"

"Well, I got really mad, actually. It was after you and I had talked that first time, you know, when you said you thought he needed an intervention? When you said you thought he was crying out for help and he needed a kick in the butt? Well, I was going along trying to work my own program, you know, not controlling, but he couldn't even get dressed by himself any more! CL, I have to help him bathe. And then I would see him, he would shoot insulin and then eat one of those pie things he likes so much. I know he's not supposed to do that. He would think I didn't know. And you know, I started to think: I am just enabling him."

"Yeah?" I urged her breathlessly.

"So, you know, he went back into the hospital the other day," Lyndsey continued. "After he had been on this so-called diet for two weeks. I got really mad. I gathered up all the cakes and cookies and stuff, stuff he had hidden all over the house – I knew where it all was, anyway – and even empty wrappers I found in the garbage and such. And I stuffed it all into a big shopping bag and I took it with me to the hospital."

I gasped. "You didn't!"

"I did," she said proudly. "And then I dumped it all on the hospital bed."

I gasped again. Imagine the shock, the horror! Imagine the guts that took. Jeeze! "You *didn't*," I exclaimed again.

"I sure did. And I told him I was tired of taking care of him when he refused to even try to take care of himself, and I wasn't going to do it any more."

"Wow!" I breathed. "Did he get mad?"

"No," she said. There is a sudden silence.

"Lyndsey?"

More silence. Then Lyndsey's voice again, choked up. "He started to cry, CL."

"Oh, my." Sudden tears sprang into my eyes.

Her voice shook a little. "He said he couldn't stop. That he was trying, but he couldn't stop cheating on the diet. And – that he was scared."

"Oh, my." My nose started dribbling and I rubbed my eyes with my sleeve and hastily peered out the bedroom door to make sure the lump of Carter was still asleep on the daybed. I didn't want him to know that we were talking about him. My throat was so tight, I had to take a few deep breaths, trying not to picture my brother in the hospital with the guilty ruins of his addiction littering the bottom of his bed, weeping, asking for help. I swallowed, staring hard at the toaster oven, trying to control myself.

"So what happened?"

"Well, I just said that he could do it," said Lyndsey. "I said I'd get rid of all the junk food in the house and he had to get the diet program up on the computer and really stick to it."

"And he agreed? I looked around and it looks like there's no junk food left in the house."

"Yes, he agreed. So, I guess he's really ready to try." She sighed happily.

"Lyndsey," I whispered, awed. "You did an intervention!"

"I did?"

"Yes, that's an intervention. Exactly."

"Well, it's all due to you," she said. "You gave me the idea."

"Maybe he'll get better now," I whispered excitedly.

"I think he will," Lyndsey whispered. "Gotta go. My boss is coming in. I'll see you later."

I wandered back into the living room and looked at my brother. He looked pretty much the same there under the old oxygen hose, his forehead red, his bowling shoulders rising and falling with each breath. I think of him scared, like my boy Byron, his eyes going wide, staring at *The Horror.*

Carter's watch alarm went off and he grabbed it with a grunt. I scurried to the kitchen to rinse my face before he could see I'd been crying.

"Cete?" he called.

"Right here."

"Time for lunch."

It was time for all of his pills and insulin, too. His watch alarm went off every couple of hours so he'd remember to take his catalog of medications. He made us a very lovely dietetic lunch: chicken salad with a yogurt-based mayonnaise, curry, and lots of celery in a hollowed out tomato on lettuce; one slice of whole grain bread cut into triangles, toasted – no butter; skimmed milk; a side salad of mesclun and baby spinach with a tahini-style dressing; and a baked apple made with Sugar Twin, cinnamon, and five raisins. He sat in a large office chair with roller wheels and did all the cooking sitting down, rolling back and forth between the fridge and the counter and the stove. As he prepared lunch, he told me about all of the ingredients and his diet computer program and how it all worked. It sounded incredibly complicated and tedious, entering recipes and calories and carbo/fat values for each ingredient.

"But once it's all in there, then you can mix and match your meals," he said excitedly. "You can have snacks. You can have desserts. You just have to make sure it's balanced. It's really not supposed to be a diet, I mean, like a short-term thing. It's supposed to be a whole system for your eating patterns, you know, changing your eating patterns for life."

"Does it count the calories?" I asked. Since I was pretty small, I already knew I can have only about 1000 to 1200 calories a day to really lose weight. Unless I could spend about two hours on the treadmill. I wondered if there are any recipes for zero-calorie fudge brownies.

"Sure," said Carter. "I'm afraid you can only have about 1,600 calories a day with moderate activity. I'm on 3,000, and that's with no activity, like I said."

"Three thousand calories a day?" I was deeply skeptical. How can anybody lose weight on 3,000 calories a day? I had a feeling he was pulling another fast one, like at the weight-loss clinic. "How can you lose weight on 3,000 calories a day?"

"It's not that much, really, when you add it all up. And I lost another two pounds. I just weighed myself this morning." He seemed so pleased with himself. He really did not appear to be cheating. At any rate, *he* believed he was doing the diet honestly.

"That's really great, Carter. It's great that you've started on a new diet."

"Yeah, well, Lyndsey and I had a little talk," he said, not looking me in the eye. "When I was in the hospital. I think I had just kind of given up, but she really inspired me to keep trying."

I pictured Lyndsey dumping his clandestine food stash on his hospital bed with a look of grim determination – I'd be inspired, too, if I were he.

"So, what can I do to help, Carter?" I asked him. "Is there anything?"

He told me he'd been wanting to try to go to the swimming pool at a recreation center in the next town. "If I can get a little exercise, it will really help take some weight off," he said. But he was worried that he wouldn't be able to get his pressure socks back on after swimming, so he didn't want to go alone.

Then he began to equivocate because I didn't have a bathing suit with me. I was so delighted that there seemed to be something I could actually do to help him, I agreed to take one of Lyndsey's bathing suits.

Since Lyndsey was almost a foot taller than I and about four sizes bigger, I did not intend to actually wear the bathing suit, but I took it along, just in case. It turned out it was a good thing I did.

It took Carter about five minutes to get down the six steps to his front door. He had to sit on the top step for a while before he got back up and took the other steps to the landing and out the door. I was not sure why he rested on the top step, since he hadn't really gone anywhere yet. Getting his courage up? You must need courage to go on.

There were twelve steps inside Carter's house. Six go from the living room to the landing where the front door is, and six more go to the lower level of the house, which was built into the side of a steep hill that sloped down toward the lake. Carter rarely went into the lower level of his house any more, where the guest room and Lyndsey's big Song Room were. He could go down the steps. It was getting back up that was the problem.

I tried to imagine what it was like to have your body fail you like this. I remembered a time when he single-handedly carried an old, queen-sized Castro-convertible couch on his shoulder up five flights of stairs. I was moving into my first apartment. My boyfriend was supposed to be helping, but the stairs were so steep and narrow, the boyfriend ended up just pulling at the top end of the antique behemoth while the weight of all that steel and wood crushed down on my brother's shoulder. I remember Carter's head cocked unnaturally to the side, away from the gold brocade, his face flushed dark red, and me fluttering around on the top landing, squeaking, "Help him, Danny! Help him!" Carter bore upward, grim and silent, one slow step at a time, till he reached the top. Now taking one step down with empty hands overwhelms his spirit with exhaustion.

It must be terrifying, I thought. It must be humiliating for him. But isn't that the beginning and the end of it all? Where human spiritual problems begin and end, I mean? Pride and humiliation. Self-esteem and self-hate. Pride that is so false it curls around and bites you in the back. Self-hatred so fierce it begs for a moving target.

Perhaps this humiliation would finally help Carter find his own "sobriety," I thought. Perhaps he had finally hit bottom. Because only through humility, said Bill Wilson, the founder of Alcoholics

Anonymous, could you come to true sobriety.

My father never could get that humility part of AA. Pop always used to ask: "But what's the difference between *humility* and *humiliation*?" Sure, humility seemed like a good thing. Humility was understanding that you are not the Big Kahuna of the Universe. Understanding that you cannot and even should not control everything. Allowing other people to help you and guide you. Admitting that the substance you abused has defeated you. All that was fine, my father thought. But how do you avoid humiliation? *Humiliation* isn't a good thing, right? Humiliation is bad. It sure feels bad. Surely Bill Wilson and Alcoholics Anonymous did not expect sobriety to result in humiliation. In fact, humiliation was awful, a torture, and ... well ... so humiliating.

Much later, after it was too late to tell my father, I figured out this much: There's not that much difference between humility and humiliation, except attitude. Humiliation is the fall from false pride, the idealized self. Bang, it hurts. Humility is gladness to be on the ground. Humiliation looks back toward false pride, at the idealized self, and feels the sneer of the universe. Humility feels the presence of all the other humans around you, looks down at the grassy ground, and finds it good.

The only tough thing was, in order to get to humility, you had to go through the humiliation. That was the thing Pop couldn't understand. You had to be willing to walk through the fire, to survive it sober and to let it crisp off the curly ribbon and crepe paper till all that was left was the naked, first version of you.

Of course, some wonderful and lucky people grew up with that honest appreciation of their true place in the universe. Right? They didn't have to struggle. Who knows, maybe even most people were that way! Just because I didn't happen to personally know any of these people, that didn't mean they didn't exist, right? Maybe you knew some of them. Me, I knew good people who struggled to be right-sized; well-intentioned people who thought they were humble but weren't; sad people who were much more humble than they should be; arrogant people who never achieved humility and didn't care; and bad people who would go to any lengths to avoid being humbled by anyone or anything.

That's the way it seemed, anyway. All I knew for sure was this: If you started out in a screwed-up alcoholic starstruck depressive obsessive-compulsive overly intellectual household, you were probably slated for trouble.

At the rec center, Carter jumped into the deep end of the Olympic-sized swimming pool, and the ripples reached me at the other end, where I was sweating in my jeans and fuzzy angora sweater. Nobody else was there at 2:45 on a Wednesday afternoon in the town of Something-ham, Massachusetts. The smell of chlorine and old feet permeated my hair. What would happen if Carter had a heart attack in the swimming pool? What was I going to do, throw him one of those inflatable whoopee-cushions big enough for him to fall on his face in? Lasso him and hitch him up to the scooter and drag him out?

Then, just as I was beginning to panic, I thought of something even more dire. Even if nothing bad happened, *how was he going to get out of the pool?* Climb the ladder? He couldn't even walk down two steps in his own house!

"Carter," I shouted with a wave.

He was standing in the deep end, the water up around his shoulders. He wiped his eyes and gave a wave, puffing. He did not waste his breath with talk.

"I changed my mind," I shouted. "I'm coming in."

I dashed into the ladies locker room and threw off my clothes. Lyndsey's one-piece bathing suit hung on me like a deflated party balloon. The part where the shoulder straps continued on down my breasts to my stomach might have been sexy were it not for the bottom half swinging down around my knees, where I was lucky my breasts (which also looked like deflated party balloons) were not also hanging after their traitorous Playboy promise of early milky motherhood.

Always the mother of invention, I whipped the straps into knots and cinched the waist with the plastic bag, which, folded twice, served as an admirable belt. I trotted back to the pool and jumped in, clutching the suit to myself as I did. Carter was still standing in the same place, his hands floating lightly on the water top. I was gripped with remorse. I should never have brought him here. He was too sick; he was trying to do too much.

But he flashed a big grin at me as I swam up holding onto a kickboard. He seemed to be feeling okay. The long jagged scar down his chest had faded with time, and wasn't so noticeable any more. I kicked unenthusiastically. I didn't really want to exercise my legs, but I thought the kickboard might come in handy in an emergency.

Maybe he had a secret method of getting out of the swimming pool, I thought. I decided I wouldn't mention the pickle we were in yet, and just exercise along with him.

"So what are we going to start with?" I said instead.

"Start what?" said Carter.

"Exercising."

"I am exercising. I'm exercising already."

"What are you doing?" I looked down through the water to see if maybe he was doing leg lifts under there.

"I'm standing!"

He laughed his rumbly belly laugh, the greatest laugh ever made. It sort of starts out in his belly and builds up into this great burbling breathless rasp that goes on and on. It was hard not to laugh when Carter was laughing. I gave a stupid little giggle. He wiggled his fingers on top of the water, then held them still, then wiggled them again.

"And these are my arm extensions," he said, wiggling his fingers again.

"Ha, ha," I said, lifting my leg to the surface and wiggling my toes. "These are my toe extensions."

Unfortunately, Carter tried to lift his leg to the surface also, and he immediately sank with a large swirl of bubbles and foam.

My reflexes were hair-trigger. "Help!" I screamed. Of course, I'd forgotten that nobody could hear us down here. The echo bounced off the chlorinated tiles.

I dove under and saw Carter smiling like a Buddha, his eyes squeezed tight shut, still tumbling back, his long, fine hair waving upward: *Goodbye, goodbye everyone.* Was he laughing or grimacing? I couldn't tell. I swam behind him and grabbed under his arms. He uncurled, and we both rose to our feet.

He panted shallow, raspy pants, wiping the water from his face.

Then he started to laugh again. Then he couldn't catch his breath because he was laughing and he panted again.

"Jesus, Carter," I said, appalled.

"Well," he panted, "that's probably enough exercise for today."

"How we gonna get out of here?" I looked around the huge pool. The stress of the moment had made me forget to be diplomatic.

"The ladder's right there," panted Carter with a nod.

Since I didn't want to say, "Yeah, but you can't climb it," I just stood there. After a while, Carter moved toward the ladder, one slow step at a time. He rested for a while once he reached it. Then he grabbed the sides of the ladder as high up as he could reach. Pulling knees to chest, he settled both feet on the second-from-the-bottom rung. I held my breath. With one powerful surge, he pushed upward through the pool, lifting off into the terrible gravity, the heavy water curling off his body like breakers off an ocean liner. His fingers clenched the ladder mightily, his knees like cold pistons reaching down into themselves for the pressure to rise, a weight-lifter's single note of effort singing out of his lips in a swelling "*Ahhhhh….*"

For a moment, I feared his trajectory would be up, up, and over, crashing back down into the pool with a sickening slap, or that the very roots of the ladder would grind out of the cement with a horrible screech and the aluminum steps would fall back into the pool on top of him.

But no – he steadied. He was holding, his body straight, his head bowed, his feet still on the second-from-the-bottom rung. The echo of his labored breathing caromed around our heads.

Slowly, he turned his head and looked at me. That look said everything. He knew very well I was afraid that he would not be able to climb the ladder, because he, also, was afraid he was not going to be able to climb the ladder. But here he was, pressing 400, a weight-lifter again! That look said: *See I didn't need that stupid kickboard! Do you think I didn't know what you were up to with that?* The look said: *See, I'm not defeated yet.* I gave him the thumbs-up and he wiggled his eyebrows, the only muscles currently not in use. Then he proceeded up the other steps, resting for a while after each one, until he had achieved the edge of the pool, where he sat down on his scooter. I re-secured my plastic-bag belt and followed him up the ladder.

"Well," I said, grabbing my towel, "that was refreshing!"

I know he would have laughed, but he was too tuckered out. His head was hanging down and his hands were on his knees, as if he could barely stay sitting upright. I scurried into the men's locker room and got his towels and his clothes, wrapped him in the towels he'd brought and then put mine around him, too. He was beginning to turn blue and quiver a little, but claimed he was just chilly. Alarmed, I kept working faster and faster. Dry his legs and feet off, scooch the pressure socks up onto his feet and roll them up his legs, get his shirt and sweatshirt on him. It was not much different from dressing a big baby, only I couldn't lay him down on the changing table. I tried to press the water out of his swim trunks and I stuck his feet into the legs of his pants. He managed to struggle into the rest of his clothes and I raced back into the ladies locker room and threw on my own clothes. I was not sure why I was racing, or exactly what I was racing against, but I felt very strongly that I had better go as fast as I could. Carter drove his scooter into the hall; I raced ahead to call the elevator. Carter maneuvered out the front door of the rec center, and I raced ahead with the keys to get the car. The more he slumped, the more I raced. I pulled up with the car and Carter drove the scooter onto the platform. He was driving with his head down so low, I wondered how he could see.

"I'll drive home," I said to Carter. "I know the way now."

He didn't object. He'd never let me drive his car before, and I gunned it as soon as we were out on Route 1, but he didn't say a thing. His chin was on his chest and his shoulder was slumped against the car-door window. His hands lay still and open on his lap, like two great conch shells.

Then he mumbled something.

"What?" I questioned loudly, as if being loud might bring some stability to the situation.

"Don't let me fall asleep," he said a little louder.

"No, ha, ha," I laugh. I sounded like a hyena. "Why, are you afraid I'll get bored?"

"Sleep apnea," he said. He cleared his throat, "I'm supposed to have my oxygen."

Then I remembered that the whole reason he slept with the oxygen was because of the sleep apnea. When Carter fell asleep, his whole body said, "Hey, bro, I thought we were getting some *rest* here" and just stopped breathing altogether. It was not uncommon, especially in obese people, and it caused things like snoring. But for Carter, it could cause a heart attack, so he couldn't sleep without the oxygen.

"Sing!" I said loudly. Then I started us off with one of the songs we used to sing in the car when we were kids, taking interminable car trips to whatever summer stock theater my father might be working in next:

Oh, the Lord he made a Garden so fair.
Dem bones gonna rise again.

"Come on, sing, Carter. Sing along!" I urged.

And then He made Adam and he put him in there.
Dem bones gonna rise again.
I knowd it Lordy, 'deed I knowd it, Brother,
I knowd it, wheee, dem bones gonna rise again.

Carter was not participating, so I shook his arm.
"Mmm," jerked Carter.
"You were sleeping," I said. "Sing with me."

He took a rib from Adam's side...
Dem bones gonna rise again.

Carter mumbled as if drugged.

And then He made Eve for to be his bride ....

He sang a few words here and there, then died out. I kept shaking his shoulder to get him started again, like a radio you keep having to adjust. "*Apples, peaches, pears and such,*" he sang in his raspy tenor, eyes closed. "*Dem bones gonna rise again,*" I responded. "*Of these fruits you dasn't touch,*" he continued after a pause. I pounded my left foot on the floor to the vigorous beat and sang really loud. I was feeling really wide awake, man! *"I knowd it, Lordy, deed I knowd it, brother ..."* I loved this song, even though I probably didn't sing it the way all those poor people must've sung it in the cotton fields, when all they had to look forward to was Armageddon.

By the time we were approaching his house, we were at the end of the great fall of humanity, and I had to shake Carter harder to wake him up. *Adam you must leave this place*, God told him. *And earn your bread by the sweat of your face.* It seemed like a harsh sentence for just eating a little apple, but then, once you *know* you are in paradise, I guess it just isn't paradise any more. We humans are just too prone to say things like, "I think you should move that apple tree over by the fence," and "Adam, why don't you dig the potatoes up *this* way!" and "Well, is this all there is?"

Once we were parked, I ran around to Carter's side and wrapped his arm around my shoulders, more to pull him along than anything else. He seemed to come more awake again, and we managed to get into the house. He did not sit down on the steps that go up to the living room, but gripped the railings and slowly hauled himself up. I thought he was afraid that if he sat, he wouldn't be able to get up again.

From there it was just a few steps to his daybed and the oxygen machine, and we took them together haltingly. He sat heavily, with a grunt, then rolled back onto the bed and held out his hand, I was guessing for the oxygen, so I handed him the plastic mask. He fiddled with something on the mask and put it on. Then he held out his hand again, but this time I didn't know what he wanted. His eyes were closed.

"What, Carter?" I said, coming closer. "What do you need?" He opened his eyes and smiled at me, grabbed my hand and patted my arm with the other hand.

"Thanks," he whispered. "That was fun."

SIXTEEN: CAN'T SOMEBODY ELSE DO ALL THIS?
April

*W*E were both asleep when Lyndsey got home from work. "Oh, my God," she said, "did you guys sleep the whole day?"

"Oh, no," I assured her, rolling off the couch with a groan, "we had an adventure."

Carter woke up. It was weird, but he seemed to be fine again. He regaled Lyndsey with the story of our rec center visit, making it sound a little less dangerous and much more silly than it was. Later, as she was preparing her dinner and Carter was preparing our dinner, she murmured to me that there was a message on the machine for me.

"One of the OA people," she said. "A guy. He said he'd be there."

Then she looked at me, eyebrows raised, a question in her eyes, but we couldn't conspire right in front of Carter, so I said, "Carter, I'm planning to go to an OA meeting around here tonight. Is that okay?"

Carter looked up from the wok. He was making a curried chicken vegetable stir-fry with homemade noodles, rolling around the kitchen on his roller chair. "Really?" he said.

"Yeah, you know, I started going at home, remember I told you? There's a meeting just in the next town over, Mattingham. That's close, right?"

"Mattingham?" said Lyndsey. "You mean Matterly?"

"That's it."

"Yeah," said Lyndsey. "That's only ten minutes."

"This sounds like a really good meeting," I said to Carter. "No gray sheet."

He looked surprised. "No gray sheet?"

"Nope. They despise gray sheet. They say gray sheet people are Nazis."

"Hmph," said Carter.

"Gee," said Lyndsey, "I didn't know there were any non-gray-sheet meetings around here."

"Yeah, there're actually quite a few."

"Hmph," said Carter, putting the food on the table.

As our delicious diet dinner was drawing to a close, I looked at my watch pointedly. "Gee, it's almost seven. The meeting starts at seven-thirty. I better get ready." Then I said casually, "Anybody want to come with me?"

"Hmph," said Carter.

"Do you know how to get there?" asked Lyndsey.

"Yeah, they gave me directions. I just go on Route One to Main Street and turn right. It's in Christ the King church on Main Street, in the church basement. They said you can't miss it."

"Yeah, but you have to be careful on Route One," said Lyndsey. "There's a traffic circle that's a little confusing. Make sure you continue on Route One after the traffic circle and don't go off on Route One-A."

"Oh, okay," I suppressed a tiny surge of irritation. "Doesn't anybody want to come with me?"

"Well, I might go," said Lyndsey, looking at her watch. Lyndsey tended toward heavy, but she was usually pretty good about sticking to her diet. She didn't really need OA.

"Oh, all right," said Carter with a sigh. "I'll go."

"Oh, that's great, Carter." I said. "That's really great. Thanks."

He began to laugh and he looked at Lyndsey, who was smiling. "I hate to make you go for nothing."

"What do you mean?" I was all innocence.

He gave me a look. He knew I was going to the OA meeting just for him.

"I think it's really going to be a good meeting, Carter!" I was grinning. I was ecstatic. Carter was going to OA. Carter was going to be saved! All my work was coming to fruition! And he even knew that I was trying to manipulate him! And he thought it was funny. That meant something didn't it? Didn't that mean that he knew he needed help? Didn't that mean he knew I was trying to save him because I loved him? Hurrah! Carter was going to be saved! I grinned like the Cheshire cat.

"You don't have to go, Lyndsey," he said. He put his arm around her waist. "You must be tired."

"Well …" Lyndsey hesitated. Should she or shouldn't she? Show support or crawl under the covers? Encourage him, or be selfish? Responsibility, or relaxation? Fear, or trust? Encouraging, or enabling? And hey, folks, what about *me*, said Lyndsey's other voice. I've been working all day, you know, what about *me*?

"Lyndsey," I told her, "we'll be fine. Just relax." I figured if Carter and I could get through the swimming pool adventure, we could get through anything.

So Carter and I got back in his car and set out for the King's basement in Matterly, Massachusetts.

First of all, Jeff, the OA member I had spoken to on the phone, met us at the door. He was actually waiting for us to show up. He warmly shook Carter's hand and welcomed him, and that made Carter feel great. There was nothing like a smile and a welcome; it did such wonders for the soul. Carter couldn't go in the regular way because there were steps going down to the basement, but it all worked out okay because he could scooter back to the parking lot, which sloped down a hill, and there was another door to the basement that was on level with the ground.

Inside, there were chairs around two long tables pushed together. Other people were coming in and filling up the chairs. They moved over to make room for Carter's scooter and said hello to Carter and to me. These people looked vibrant. Their faces glowed; their step was quick. They chatted and laughed. There was a happy buzz in the room, a healthy energy. Some of the people were obese, but many of them looked completely normal. There were more women than men, but at least there *were* men – seven of them – and they ranged in age from a young fellow in earrings who looked barely out of his acne years to a gentleman in a Ralph Lauren Polo shirt with white hair and an athletic build.

The meeting was led by a woman named Doris who introduced

herself as a "recovering compulsive overeater," and in unison everybody said, "Hi, Doris!" I nearly jumped off my chair. It sounded like a football stadium cheer.

Doris read something that told everybody what OA was all about and described what this meeting would be like. "There are no specific requirements for a plan of eating," she read. You could tell they'd had some trouble with gray sheet meetings around here. "OA does not endorse, recommend or distribute any specific food plan, nor does it exclude the personal use of one."

I sneaked a look at Carter. Was this sinking in? Did he get it? This was exactly what he'd been looking for! I couldn't really see his face though. He was turned toward the speaker.

"For specific dietary or nutritional guidance," Doris continued to read, "OA suggests consulting a qualified health care professional, such as a physician or dietitian. The Winner's Circle meeting is a one-hour speaker/discussion meeting. A speaker will share about his or her experience, strength, and hope for about 20 minutes, and then we will have an open discussion with a show of hands. Is there anyone celebrating an anniversary of a year or more this month?"

Several hands shot up and Doris called on them one by one. "My name is Michael, I'm a recovering compulsive overeater, and yesterday I celebrated two years of abstinence."

The room burst into applause for Michael. Several others also celebrated anniversaries of five, three, and two years of abstinence, and one of them also identified herself as a recovering alcoholic as well as a compulsive overeater, and she was celebrating seven years of sobriety *and* abstinence. This was great, I thought. This was really going to show Carter that this program worked. I was already picturing Carter walking around with these other OA folks, free from his scooter, his body strong again, his face glowing with health and happiness. I was dying to get a look at his face right now, to see how he was taking all of this in. I wanted to give him a little poke to make him turn around, but I'd have to lean way over to do so. On his scooter, he was too far away for me to murmur anything confidential, either.

After anniversaries, Doris asked, "Is anybody new to OA or new to this meeting who would like to identify themselves?"

Carter's hand, one among many, shot up immediately. I was thrilled that he was participating. Doris called on one of the obese women sitting toward the front.

"Hi, I'm Nona," she said. "This is my first time at this meeting."

"Hi, Nona," roared everyone, with various cries of "Welcome" and "Keep coming."

Hands shot up again, including Carter's. I raised my hand, too. Doris called on the woman sitting next to Nona and obviously friends with her. She was an attractive, dark-skinned Indian woman dressed in a golden caftan.

"Hi, I'm Sandra," said Nona's friend. "This is my first time at this meeting."

Again, the crowd roared a welcome, this time to "Sandra."

Then Doris called on Peter on the other side of the table, and then she called on me.

But Carter had begun shaking his arm each time he lowered it, as if it were uncomfortable. Shake, jiggle, flop-flop. It was his right arm, the heart arm. Did it hurt? Was it hard for him to hold it up in the air like that? When Doris called on me, I wanted to jump up and say, "Call on my brother. I'm giving my turn to my brother!" I could tell he was getting uncomfortable, or worse yet, annoyed. It couldn't be possible that Doris was specifically avoiding him! But it was unfortunate, I thought, that she called on everyone else around Carter without calling on him yet.

I recognized this as a familiar anxiety, and suddenly I remembered taking Harry to baby gymnastics when he was three and a half, and how they made the children raise their hands and wait their turns before they could get onto the giant trampoline and pretend to be popcorn. All the other kids seemed to be able to do this, but it drove Harry into the screaming meemies every single time he had to wait. It must be something genetic, I thought. People in our family were just constitutionally incapable of waiting their turn.

Even so, I did not jump up and say "Call on my brother, he's dying," but meekly mentioned my name and the fact this was my first time at this meeting *and* only my second OA meeting, to which the room responded with a resounding hello and welcome and "keep coming."

Carter did not raise his hand again, but Doris called on him anyway. He was the last one.

"Hi, I'm Carter," he said. "I'm a compulsive overeater and I'm probably every other kind of addict too, and this is the first time I've ever been at a real OA meeting around here. I've been to other OA meetings in Bentham and in Natterly, and in those meetings you have to go by this gray sheet diet or you're not allowed to speak." He radiated an angry energy. I couldn't see his face, but I could feel it rising off his shoulders like steam, percolating into the room. "It seems to me that from what you said at the beginning of the meeting that those other meetings shouldn't even be allowed to call themselves OA!"

I could sense other people around me beginning to shift uncomfortably as Carter spoke. Why the heck couldn't he just do the same as everybody else? Say his name and be done with it? Why did he have to make a speech? Why did he have to be different? Being different was a matter of pride in our family. We were so different we couldn't even fit into a group of people who were *all* different. I'd spent half my life trying to figure out how to fit in. Why did Carter insist on blowing it this way?

"I went to one meeting where I tried to talk about the diet I was given at Systems House …"

"Thank you, Carter," said Doris, interrupting him. "We don't do gray sheet here, and you can share after the speaker, when there's a show of hands." She turned and went on quickly, "We're lucky to have a wonderful speaker and a wonderful friend of mine who is going to tell her story tonight …"

There were a few voices that rose in salutation as Doris talked on. The ritual "Hi, Carter" fizzled with a couple of wimpy "Welcomes." It was nothing like the resounding roar that greeted the others. He had broken the rhythm; he had put them off their stride.

A sensation of dread filled me. I still could not see Carter's face. He had gone perfectly still, his rounded back like stone. Why did he do this, I wondered. Why was it he had to do everything his own way and not the accepted way? Why did he turn other people against him when he needed them so much?

The speaker sat at the head of the long table and began to tell her story, and after a while, I was pulled into it. The tension eased out of me. The story was absolutely riveting. It was the story of a family shattered by alcoholism, as ours was. The story of subtle messages and subterranean abuse, of cruelty mixed with love, of sexual abuse by an uncle, and of an older sister who fought him and won. It was a story of taking consolation in food, escaping through food, treating oneself with food, being loved by food, a story of secrets and of shame. It was a story of recovery, too, of courage and honesty and hope. The tears sprang to everyone's eyes as she talked about her sister's eventual suicide, and everyone laughed and cheered as she talked about her own stumbling start in OA and the growing strength of her spiritual, emotional, and physical program. She was celebrating eight years of abstinence. At the end of her talk, another woman sitting near her, whom she thanked as her sponsor, jumped up and embraced her.

Immediately after she had finished speaking, my hand was waving in the air along with a dozen others. When I was called on, I gushed. "Oh, I was raised in an alcoholic family, too, and I've done that very same thing that you talked about, eating sweets for consolation, or to give myself a 'treat' because I'm feeling so sad and sorry for myself."

Carter had turned to look at me with a stolid but interested expression, and my enthusiasm waxed hotter, my effort to explain what I was feeling more intense, as if Carter might be cured if I could express it well enough, if I could just convey my appreciation and understanding to him in a huge wave of words that would break over him like a christening and leave him renewed. I went on about how moving her story was, how my brother and I were here for the first time, and how wonderful it was to see this program work and all of the recovery in the room. About how our father got sober in AA before he died, and how wonderful that program was, and how grateful I was that there was OA also, and as I was saying this, tears started leaking from my eyes, even though I had no idea why. And then, to my horror, I actually *sobbed*.

It was like being in a dream where you look down and suddenly realize that you are walking around in your underwear. Oh my God, I thought as I struggled to get a grip on this runaway emotion, what was *happening* to me? How could I actually *cry* in front of all these strangers?

But everybody was so nice. A few people were patting my back. People were smiling and nodding, as if they didn't think I was at all weird. They said, "Keep coming back." Carter reached over and patted my shoulder. He was smiling again, and his glance was half glad, half concerned, his face softened with affection, and when he did that, I gave *another* little sob.

And then I realized it was about Carter – how sad I was about Carter. How much tension I'd been carrying, like holding my breath. And all of a sudden it seemed like maybe, just maybe, somebody else could shoulder the burden. Maybe somebody else could save him. Maybe I couldn't save him, but the much greater power of this group could – this ranging, electrifying joy that circled around the room like a jolt of life. This solidarity of people who came together for one purpose: to get well. To support each other in recovery from whatever it was that tortured you, from whatever it was that pulled and pushed and kicked you down that terrible road toward self-destruction; to renew the spirit and save the body; to honor each person's struggle and to demand each person's truth. It was this that made me cry, something that I had seen here, something glimpsed that was greater than myself, something that might just have the power to lift my brother from his illness and make him whole again.

When the meeting was over, a number of people crowded up to me and introduced themselves and told me to keep coming. I introduced each person to Carter, who cordially shook hands.

In the car going home, I tried to get Carter to talk about the meeting.

"It was pretty good," he admitted grudgingly. "I didn't like that woman who was in charge, though."

"Well," I said cautiously, "you know, you really weren't supposed to start talking at that point. You know, right then at the beginning, when everybody was introducing themselves? You know, when she kinda cut you off?"

"How was I supposed to know that?" Carter burst out angrily. "That's what I mean about these people. They're just into shaming you if you don't do everything their way."

"Oh, come on, Carter. These people were really nice. Nobody wanted to make you feel bad!" I did think that Doris might have been a little gentler in the way she cut him off, though. What was it about Carter? Why did he irritate people? He was so wrapped up in his own thoughts and feelings, pressed so urgently from within to tell the world what he saw, he seemed to be unaware of what was going on with the people around him. He would tread on toes and then feel hurt when people pushed him off.

When we got to the house, Lyndsey wanted to know all about the meeting. Carter chuckled and told her how much I liked the meeting. "She had this whole cathartic reaction," he said.

"Well, you liked it too, didn't you?" I said defensively.

"Sure," he said, "it was a good meeting."

"Are you going to go back?" I felt aggressive. I thought I might start to growl at him soon.

He yawned and stretched, looking away. "Oh, I don't know," he said. "Maybe."

"Please go back, Carter," I said. "It's great. Lyndsey, you have to go with him. There is so much great recovery there. The people were terrific."

"Yeah, except for the lady who runs the whole thing!" said Carter.

Suddenly, my growl vanished. I was more exhausted than I could bear. My whole body felt like a ten-ton weight. "Oh, God, I have to go to bed," I said. "I'm beat!"

I heard them murmuring about the meeting as I headed downstairs to the guest room. Just as I was sliding into the great tunnel of sleep, there was a rustle in the dark, and Lyndsey's voice. "CL?"

She was standing by the door, the light spilling from the hall, her nightgown floating around her ankles. I sat up.

"Yeah?"

She came over to me and sat on the bed and gave me a big hug. "Thank you," she whispered.

"I don't know if it did any good."

"He got more out of it than you think."

"I don't know if he'll go back."

"Even if he doesn't," she said, pressing her arms around me. "Thank you."

The tears stung my eyes again. She was such a kind and loving person. It was kind for her to be grateful, as if I had done something really useful. It had to be very hard for Lyndsey; it was terrible to feel so helpless, I thought. And then I realized, suddenly, that my tears were not for her.

SEVENTEEN: STUFFING IT, 1994 – 1996

*W*E are converging upon Mom for her birthday. Since his wedding a year ago, Carter has gotten heavier than ever. I don't understand it; he seems happy, yet he is becoming less healthy. Once he felt safe with a loving partner, he let everything go. As if, because someone else loved him, he didn't need to love himself any more.

However, he is trying to diet once again, which is a big relief to everyone. Lyndsey is very supportive. She is doing the Healthy Heart Diet together with Carter. When they get to Mom's house, they bring in a big, red ice chest full of Healthy Heart food.

I don't know Lyndsey very well. She is the child of an alcoholic, too. She fits in nicely with our family. I've met her only a few times, the second time being the wedding where she and Carter wore white beaded buckskin and sang and drummed their own, special ceremony of union. Carter makes all their meals, I hear, because Lyndsey does not like to cook. I think that might be why he's gotten heavier, but Caroline says he can't ride his bike any more because the angina has come back, and that's why he has gotten heavier. *It might have something to do with eating too much,* I say to Caroline. I hide my Girl Scout chocolate mint cookies in my suitcase and occasionally adjourn to the bedroom for a Girl Scout pick-me-up.

At dinner, Mom exhibits great restraint by making us fillet of sole and salad with lemon dressing … no biscuits, no dessert … but Carter isn't eating any of it, anyway. He cooks up a huge meal of salmon and pasta for himself and Lyndsey. In the morning, Carter gets out Mom's mixing bowl. I think maybe he is going to make Mom a birthday cake, but he fills it with three different kinds of cereal and tops it off with lots of Sweet & Low.

Back in the bedroom, Sean says in a low voice, "What is going on?"

"What?" I say innocently.

"I thought Carter was on a diet."

"He is!" I am relieved Sean has not found my Girl Scout cookies. He thinks I eat too much sugar.

"Why is he eating a *mixing bowl* of cereal?"

I shrug. "He always uses a bowl like that. It's Healthy Heart cereal."

"I don't care what kind of cereal it is! Eating a mixing bowl full of cereal every morning is not good for your heart."

I nod sagely. "Why don't you mention it to him?"

"You tell him. He's your brother."

Instead, I tell my mother. "Ma, Carter is eating too much. He ate a whole mixing bowl full of cereal for breakfast."

Mom shakes her head. "I can't tell him what to do, CL."

Later, Mom mentions it to Lyndsey. "Does he always eat that much at breakfast, Lynn?"

"Yeah," says Lyndsey. "But I'm not going to say anything about it." Lyndsey tells me the Healthy Heart diet is really exhausting. "It's so much work!" So far, Carter hasn't lost any weight.

I go back to Sean. "Lyndsey says Carter isn't losing weight. "

"You gotta tell him to eat less," says Sean.

*   *   *

Carter is arguing with the Services Director.

"One thousand calories is not enough for someone my size," insists Carter.

"Mr. Watson, we've been using a one-thousand calorie diet for all of our residents, whatever their size. It's been working really well."

Carter is half-way through his first week at Systems House, a place in Virginia where people go to lose weight. It is very expensive. Mom is paying for Carter to stay for the four-week program.

"A person my size should have at least sixteen hundred calories a day," says Carter. "A thousand calories? That's nothing! It doesn't make sense to give all different people the same diet. Here." He thrusts a clipboard full of neat columns of notes and numbers at the Services Director. "I've worked it all out."

The Services Director takes the clipboard wearily. His face is red and his blood pressure is going up. He is hot and tired. He glances at Carter's columns. "Okay. Whatever you say, Mr. Watson."

In the dining room, the other Systems House guests eye Carter's plate. "Hey, how come you get more?" they ask.

Carter explains why he should get more than everyone else. He shows them his chart. Some of the others shake their heads and mutter to each other.

"I can see your point," says one man, who doesn't even look overweight to Carter. "But it might be better to do it the way everybody does it."

Carter shrugs and his face gets stiff. "I think my way makes sense."

"This place is torture," Carter tells Lyndsey. "Everybody is really unfriendly."

"Hang in there," she tells him. At the end of three weeks, he leaves the program and goes home to Lyndsey. He has lost thirty-five pounds and he is feeling much better.

Over the next two months, he will gain all the weight back.

*   *   *

It is Thanksgiving, and we all meet at Mom's house. I am worried about Carter eating too much. I have heard that he now has diabetes, brought on by the obesity.

Caroline and I discuss it on the phone.

"We've got to make some non-sugar stuff," I say. "I'll make a non-sugar pie and we can make the sweet potatoes without sugar."

But when I get there, Carter has brought his own version of Mom's traditional sweet potato casserole, thick with brown sugar and raisins and butter and marshmallows, and Mom has pumpkin pies and pecan pies (with whipped cream for us and ice cream for the boys), as well as the turkey and the stuffing and the rolls and homemade biscuits and corn pones with honey and corn and rice and gravy with giblets and creamed spinach and peas and sautéed carrots and salad. Where Mom is from, a meal is a meal is a meal. O, it is divine! As always. A feast to leave everybody groaning!

Except Carter. Carter isn't groaning. Carter is sweating.

"Is this *caffeinated* tea?" he demands, snatching his hand back from the frosty, foaming iced tea glass as he finishes a swig and lands the glass next to his knife.

"Uh, it might be. I'm not sure," I volunteer, jumping up to check the instant iced tea mix in the kitchen. Mom jumps up, too.

"There's decaf, I'll get it, I'll get it," she says.

"Jesus Christ, you'll give me a heart attack," Carter mutters in an undertone to nobody in particular. I think it is pretty mean to say that, but actually I am surprised that my mother has made all of this food. Why wasn't she more careful? Carter has not been allowed to have caffeine ever since his heart attack.

The instant iced tea mix stands in two jars, side by side, one decaf and the other caff. Nobody knows which is in Carter's glass, so he gets a new one, and the meal goes on. Carter, whose hors d'oeuvre was a big dose of insulin, piles his plate high with everything and eats it all down to the china. In our time-honored family tradition, nobody says a word. And in another time-honored family tradition, we all have pieces of each and every pie lathered with whipped cream, including my surprisingly tasty non-sugar apple pie. Carter also helps the children ladle out their ice cream, graciously consenting to judge the relative merits of Chocolate-Chip Cookie Dough, Harry's favorite, versus Byron's favorite, Deep Devil Chocolate Fudge (a choice which, it must be admitted, is influenced more by Byron's attraction to the language than by the inherent superiority of the ice cream. I know this because after eating several desserts of my own, I also graciously consent to judge between the two ice creams.)

Uncle Carter, always wonderfully jolly and fun with children, judges both ice creams The Best, and sits heavily down on the couch facing the sunroom's extra-big dinner table.

The children start crawling all over him as usual, expecting him to toss them up in the air like beach balls, where they can squeal and revolve and generally gratify their antigravitational, me-centric desires. But Carter is having none of it.

"I can't do it now," he says for the second time, growing angry. His big, soft face is blanched to the color of wallpaper paste.

"Harry, Byron, leave Uncle Carter alone now," I say, frightened.

They begin to protest. Carter leans back against the couch. Sweat trickles down the sides of his face and he is breathing like an engine. "Lyndsey, get my kit," he says.

I grab the kids by their wrists and roughly drag them to their feet. "Stop it! Stop it!" I shout. "Go inside." The boys just stand there.

"Harry, Byron!" Sean says angrily. "Listen to your mother."

They ignore him, too, agog.

Lyndsey hands Carter his diabetes kit, a compact zip-up lunchbox of drugs and needles. Lyndsey doesn't seem rattled. I figure she's seen this before. I stare hard at her calm face, trying to read what is happening to Carter, my mouth having fallen into a little o.

"Come on, boys." Caroline sweeps by to the rescue. "Let's build the Lego spaceship."

"We can play later," Carter says to the boys with a lame smile. "I just have to rest now."

They trot like puppies after Caroline toward the living room. "Is Uncle Carter having a heart attack?" Byron's voice drifts back.

"Byron, be quiet!" hisses his elder brother, having already learned the family code of silence.

Lyndsey and my mother wheel in Carter's breathing machine. It is a big cabinet with a fat, plastic hose coming out of it.

"Is he going to be all right?" I murmur to Lyndsey.

She glances at him, cool as a nurse. He's pricked his finger and is testing his blood. "Yeah, he's okay. I think he needs some more insulin."

Since he has to take his pants off to shoot the insulin into his thigh, I leave the room. Later, I go back in to take a peek at him. He is lying on his side under a blanket, asleep, the breathing mask held in place with elastic bands that go behind his head. I wonder how he can sleep with that thing on his face, but he's been using it for a few years now for the sleep apnea. Without the breathing machine, the sleep apnea might make Carter have another heart attack.

I see Lyndsey talking to my mother in the kitchen in quiet tones. Lyndsey is crying. I don't want to go in there. Emma is reading magazines in her room. In the back, Caroline is still helping the kids build their Lego toys. If I show my face, I'll have to play too, so I don't want to go there, either. Sean is taking a nap in the bedroom. Naps are good. Napping is definitely where I'd rather be. You don't have to think or worry when you nap. I snuggle down into the covers with Sean and consign myself to oblivion.

*   *   *

The social worker from the hospital calls Lyndsey. "Mrs. Watson, has your husband ever been diagnosed with psychological problems?"

Carter is in the hospital overnight to stabilize his blood sugar. Lyndsey is expecting him home the following day.

She is taken aback by the nurse's question. "Uh, I don't know. He was taking Prozac when I met him, but he stopped taking it. Why, what's going on?"

"I've been asked to help," says the social worker. "He seems very angry and it is difficult to get him to comply with the doctor's instructions."

"Oh," says Lyndsey. She dreads the whole thing. She doesn't want to get involved. "Well," she admits, "he doesn't like being told what to do."

"He needs to do what he is told," says the social worker. "How else can we help him?"

"Sure," says Lyndsey, "that's true. Why don't you tell him that?"

*   *   *

Thanksgiving at Mom's was a terrible shock. I am sure Carter is about to die. I call and arrange to visit him – just me, no kids, no husband. I have decided I must confront him about his eating. But when I get there, Carter is already on a new diet. He feels optimistic about it: Someone else prepares all their food and he just eats what is there for him. It's a relief, but it's also a disappointment. Hasn't this happened before? Carter and I have a nice visit. We go to the movies. We eat his prepared diet meals. We watch TV.

I am just trying to say goodbye when Carter comes out of his study in tears.

"What's wrong?" I say, my stomach plummeting.

"Why did you come here?" Carter shouts at me. Carter is crying and shouting angrily at the same time, what I privately call *"krouting."* Krouting is one of those things that happens a lot in dysfunctional families.

"I wanted to see you!" I try shouting back, without much success. My voice peters out. "What, is that a crime?"

"Did you come here to put me on a diet?"

My heart is pounding and my hands are shaking, but I am trying to defend myself. "You're already on a diet!"

"Did you come here to spy on me for Mom or Caroline?"

He is really furious. I can't believe he is so paranoid. "Of course not. Don't be ridiculous. If you must know, I was afraid you were going to drop dead at Thanksgiving and I wanted to see you before you went."

He stalks into the kitchen, and I can't leave without going past him. "I've been dying for the past ten years," he shouts over his shoulder. "So what's new about that?"

The self-pity is dripping from the rafters. I am sorry I ever came, and I wish I could vanish. But Lyndsey steps in to the rescue. She calms everybody down and we talk. "I'm worried about you," I tell Carter. "I don't know how to help you."

"Just be there," says Carter. "There's nothing else you can do."

EIGHTEEN: YOU ALWAYS HURT THE ONES YOU LOVE
April to September

*C*ARTER awoke in darkness. There was a weight on his chest. He tried long, slow, deep breaths, but still it felt like he had been running. He could not catch his breath.

He was not afraid, but he was concerned. The oxygen did not help. Always, there was the feeling of being caught short. He could not get enough air, as if his chest were filled with foam that pressed on his lungs and heart, as if his organs were packed into something too stiff to give. Quietly, without turning on the light, he rose from the reclining chair and slipped on his pants, his shirt, stepped into his shoes, and got his wallet from the desk in the office where the computer still glowed. His breath rattled in his own ears: a rasping in, a hesitation, a soft expostulation out. He did not want anyone to wake, and he held tight to the railing as he descended the stairs to the front door.

Lyndsey woke as the car started in the driveway. She stared a moment into the darkness, then saw the bedroom wall briefly illuminated by a sliding bar of light, the painting of irises and lilies played out in a black and white glare. Her hand reached under the covers to the other side of the bed, where it was already cold. She rolled back into the warmth, curled up around her pillow, heedless of the bright green seconds ticking by on the illuminated clock.

*   *   *

It was still dark when Lyndsey woke me up.

"I'm sorry to have to wake you."

"What's going on?"

"Carter wasn't feeling so well in the night, and he drove himself over to the hospital. He didn't want to wake anybody."

"Oh, no." I sat up with the adrenaline suddenly pumping through me. "We did too much. I shouldn't have taken him to the swimming pool."

"I don't think it's too serious," said Lyndsey, "but they decided to admit him, so he called and asked me to bring his diabetes stuff over before I go to work."

The glimmer of predawn seeped into the room through the high windows. Lyndsey was already dressed and had her coat on.

"You're leaving now?"

"Yeah, I'm sorry, I've got to go now," she said. "Do you know where all the breakfast food is?"

"Yeah, but what's the matter with him? Why did he go to the hospital?"

"He was having trouble catching his breath, he said. Even with the oxygen."

"Is he having another heart attack?" My voice quavered a little. Maybe this was it! Maybe it was all over now.

"No, no, it's not his heart. Don't worry, I don't think it's anything really bad."

"I have to go home today," I said.

"I know," said Lyndsey. "I'll call you. Don't worry."

After tossing and turning for another hour, I finally got up and hit the road. Not far from home, I managed to get through to Carter in the hospital.

"What's the matter? What happened?"

"Well," he said with an apologetic tone, "they think I might have pneumonia. I gotta stay here for a few days." His breathing was labored and he paused every so often.

"Pneumonia!"

"Yeah. I'm sorry (*puff, puff*) I didn't get to say goodbye. I didn't want to wake you up."

"Oh, my God. I should never have taken you to that swimming pool." I was stricken. Good Lord! Here I went to help him recover and I landed him in the hospital.

"Naw," Carter scoffed, puffing. "It has nothing to do with that. I had bronchitis last month, and they think maybe it never really cleared up."

"I'm so sorry; I wore you out too much."

"No, no," he insisted breathlessly. "It was great to see you. Thanks for coming to visit me. Really, Cete. I know you're trying to help me."

There was a silence. Just the sound of his breathing.

"I gotta go," he said. "The doctor's coming in."

As soon as I got home, I crashed. Sean wanted to hear all about Carter and everything that happened, but I mumbled only a few words before I fell asleep. I didn't wake up again until the children were home from school, using me as a trampoline.

"I don't think I did any good," I told Sean when we got a few minutes alone. "The OA meeting was great for me, but I don't think he'll go back."

"Lyndsey called while you were asleep," he said. "She's worried because Carter's already ordering stuff from the deli."

"God damn it! Every time he goes into the hospital, he blows it. If only I could get him into OA."

"You did what you could," said Sean. "You never know. You planted a seed."

I was depressed and my mood was not helped any by my mother's call an hour later.

"Carter's back in the hospital," she said in a controlled, upbeat voice.

"Yeah, I know."

Mom thought it was thrilling that I got Carter to go to an OA meeting, but I was pessimistic.

"It always throws him off when he goes into the hospital," I said. "Did you ever notice that? He gets going on a diet and then he goes into the hospital for something and then when he comes out, he's not on the diet any more. He starts eating bad stuff in the hospital because he hates the food there so much. You know, he orders up from that deli."

"Maybe the hospital people could sort of, you know, stick to his diet plan for his meals."

"You think they're going to do *his* diet?" I said bitterly.

"Well," said Mom. "We could ask them. He's going to be in there at least a week, they say."

"They'll do whatever it is they do. They're not going to think about him as an addict, you know. *They're* not going to try to fit into *his* program of recovery!"

"Well …" she faltered, and suddenly I felt like a mook for being so nasty. What I was really bitter about was my own failure. What did I think I was going to accomplish? An overnight miracle?

"Well, maybe you're right," I said quickly. "We could ask them. You know. Talk to his doctor."

But I never even tried to get through to his doctor. I was more than discouraged, even though I did not admit it to myself. I dragged myself through the next day. I felt I had failed. I was out of ideas. I was embarrassed that I liked the OA meeting so much and Carter didn't. We were supposed to be going for him, not me. Somewhere, I had made a mistake, but I was not sure what I did wrong. I still felt guilty about Carter ending up in the hospital, and anxiously I contemplated the future. Would Lyndsey leave him if he didn't go back on the diet? What would he do if Lyndsey left him? What would *we* do if Lyndsey left him?

Weeks passed, and then a month. I had given up. I could hardly bear to talk to Carter on the telephone. We were in the middle of the busy B&B season, and another month slipped by. I kept track of Carter's progress through Mom. It seemed like Carter was getting better, but then he was in the hospital again. Then he was back home again, on his diet and doing water aerobics at the rec center.

It was a roller coaster. First I thought he was getting well; then it seemed like he might die. First he was on his diet; then he was cheating on his diet. I felt guilty and angry at the same time. Why had Carter gotten himself into this mess in the first place? If only I had had the courage to make a scene about it at the family reunion so many years ago, when I realized he must have angina.

There must be something I could do, I thought, but I didn't know what. The more helpless I felt, the more I ignored the whole situation. Carter didn't call me, and I rarely called him. The summer dragged on, and it was not until the end of August, when I met a B&B guest named Rita, that I was inspired with a whole new plan of action.

*   *   *

Rita and Maurice showed up very late on a Friday night the weekend before Labor Day. I didn't get a good look at them until Saturday morning breakfast. They were an older couple, short, compact, and glowing with energy. Maurice was all grizzly gray and had a very clipped gray beard and sparkling hazel eyes and very white teeth. Rita was even smaller, with a pouf of red hair and skin as translucent as morning dust. They'd brought their mountain bikes with them and they were all dressed for some serious exercise.

After breakfast, Rita complemented me on the healthiness of our buffet spread. They were all dressed to go out biking and I was sitting in front of the fire drinking coffee, feeling morose. I had just spoken to Carter, who was in the hospital with bronchitis again.

"Yeah," I said, "I try to be pretty health-conscious when it comes to food."

She told me she was a nutritionist, and I told her I had a brother who was obese and very ill.

A look came over her face. "Maurice," she said, "start without me."

Maurice grinned. "She's a woman on a mission," he said. Instead of leaving, he took his jacket off and sat down with a look of anticipation. You could tell he thought Rita was the cat's meow. Rita held up a finger.

"Just one minute." She hurried back into their room and returned holding some papers and some photographs. She threw the photos onto the coffee table. "Take a look."

They were pictures of a very heavy woman, tremendously obese, almost as wide as she was tall. I gave her a questioning look.

"Me!" she said.

"No!" I looked back at the pictures. It didn't even look like her.

"Twenty years ago."

"Wow."

"Rita specializes in treating lifetime obese patients at Mount Tremper Hospital," said Maurice.

"We have a very special program," said Rita. "We treat not only the body, but also the emotions and the spirit of a person. Obesity is an addictive illness. You have to treat the whole person. More and more, the medical establishment is beginning to realize that."

Rita and I talked about Carter for an hour. I told her all about his problems and my problems and our family's problems. She told me all about the program at Mount Tremper Hospital and how it worked. Unfortunately, it was an outpatient program in New Jersey, so there was not much chance that Carter could take advantage of it. She questioned me closely about Carter's health issues and about his situation at home, and she urged me to continue to try to help him.

" It's never too late to lose weight and get healthier. You'd be amazed at the body's resilience once you begin to treat it right. It's a great first step that your sister-in-law confronted him," said Rita. "He committed himself to a reasonable diet. Now he just needs the support to get back into it when he gets out of the hospital."

"Yeah," I said, "well that's why I tried to get him into OA. But I don't think he's going to go."

"Have you tried family therapy?" said Rita.

This was a new idea. "Well, I was going to try a family intervention," I said.

"It sounds like your sister-in-law already did the intervention. At Mount Tremper, when we have a patient who shies away from groups like OA, it really helps if we begin with family therapy. That's the first, most important 'group' for the patient to get comfortable in. And if he is struggling to go back onto his diet when he gets out of the hospital, a family therapy meeting could function sort of like a soft intervention – get him going again. Maybe there are issues that still need to be worked out in your family."

"Could be," I admitted.

By the time Rita and Maurice pedaled off, I was convinced that family therapy was The Answer for Carter. I spent the afternoon in my office on the Internet, abandoning the children to their computer games until they forced me to pay attention to them.

"Mommy," said Byron as I realized that he was at once jiggling my elbow and rubbing my head in a very annoying manner, "I'm hungry."

"I'm hungry, too," said Harry.

It was that food thing again. "Did we eat lunch?" I said. It was two o'clock.

"No," they chorused.

I'd just done a very promising search and I couldn't stop right then. "There's hard-boiled eggs in the fridge," I said.

"Yuck."

"You love hard-boiled eggs."

"I hate hard-boiled eggs," said Harry.

"Since when?"

"For years now!" said Harry. "I used to like them, but I started hating them *years* ago."

The site I was searching led on to a number of accredited psychologists who did addictions counseling and family therapy. I started going through the list. "Well, there's peanut butter in the cabinet," I mumbled. "Go make yourselves some sandwiches."

"Mommy, that peanut butter is yucky."

"It's real peanut butter," I told them. "It's ground up peanuts."

"Why can't you get the good kind of peanut butter?" whined Harry, by which he meant the kind with the sugar in it.

I rounded on them with teeth bared, an inarticulate gargle in my throat, and they scampered off to the kitchen.

About twenty minutes later, my search having yielded two possible names for further investigation, I noticed something. It was very quiet. Very, very quiet. Except for an occasional, very loud *thump*. And a giggle.

Uh-oh.

I crept upstairs to the kitchen. More giggles. I crept a little faster. The door was ajar and I peered in.

There was ice cream everywhere, especially on the dog. New ice cream, old ice cream, ice cream eaten almost to the bottom of the container and then saved until fossilized, ice cream melting in small puddles on the floor. Ice cream on the cabinets. Ice cream on the dog's ears. Ice cream in Byron's hair. Ice cream paw prints on the linoleum. A gallon of chocolate ice cream melting on the table. A container of Cookies 'n Cream that must be twenty years old leaking onto the counter. An empty Haagen Dazs pint container of Macadamia Nut on the chair. A very old Ben and Jerry's Chocolate Chip Cookie Dough container lying on its side by the stove. Byron was riding on top of Rue, who was chasing Harry, who was running in a circle around the central island counter, holding a large spoon of ice cream.

"Ha," shouted Harry, turning and flinging the ice cream at Byron.

"Ha, ha," shouted Byron, whirling ice cream from atop his steed. Rue twisted in an impossible pretzel trying to catch both flings of ice cream in his mouth at the same time, and Byron fell to the floor. *Thump.*

I went crazy. There's no other word for it. My mind slipped into that terrible pit inside of me, and a helpless twist of fury lacerated my consciousness.

"What's the meaning of this!" I screamed. "Who do you think you are?" Which was what my father used to say. But I was not thinking about my father. My mind was boiling: *These kids have no respect!* And, *Never any time for myself!* And, *Where the hell is Sean!* Thoughts lashed me: *We will never have enough money to help Carter,* and, *This is out of control,* and, *What a lousy mother I am!* Frustration gonged in my head. Rage blazed through my pipes like wild fire. My throat roughened and burned.

"How dare you do such a thing!" I screamed. "This is our home. This is our business. We have guests here!" Actually, there were no guests in the house at the moment, or I wouldn't have been screaming. Harry crouched on the floor, bunched up into a knot, his hands over his ears. He looked like he was riding out a blitz. Byron was half-reclining, like Laura in Oliver Winslow Homer's painting, a dramatic look of horror on his face. Rue was cowering with his ears back, licking the floor as fast as he could.

Then something really bad happened. Byron giggled. He glanced over at Harry and giggled again, and I could see his amusement infecting Harry, who so far had been properly cowed. I threw myself on my knees in front of Byron, outraged.

"You think it's funny?" I shouted, pushing my face close up to his. "You think this is FUNNY?"

He reached a finger toward my forehead, still struggling against giggles. "It's just you have a …"

I did not find out what I had on my face because my rage had reached the flash point. Maybe it was because his finger invaded my space, that final, sheer barrier of air between what was his and what was mine.

Maybe it was because I was abused when I was a child. Maybe it was because he would not be dominated by me. Maybe it was because I was mad, and I knew I could get away with it. Whatever. I *kapowed*, like magnesium under a match. I *whooshed*. Everything went white. My hand flew up, knocking Byron's hand aside, and I slapped his face good and hard, hard enough to rock him backward, hard enough to leave four red marks on his pale, petal-like cheek.

Immediately, I felt horrible. There was a wolf tearing at my heart. The shame. The error. The cruelty. I knew it was wrong, and so did Byron. He looked at me with disbelief, his face crumpling.

"You said you'd *never* do that again!" he said, his fingers going to his cheek.

"I'm so sorry, Byron."

He twisted the knife. "You *lied*."

I had done it before, exactly the same way, before I knew what was happening, driven by a flash of rage. I had promised myself and him I would never slap his face again, and here I was, once again out of control.

"How could you be so disrespectful?" I said, dismayed. I groped for reasons. That old song came into my head, *"You always hurt the one you love..."*

"Mommy," said Harry, pulling at my sleeve.

"You lied!" Byron repeated, holding his cheek, his eyes blazing. Then the tears come flooding down. Sobs. Such grief as you could die from.

"Mommy," said Harry, tapping me.

"I'm sorry I slapped your face again, Byron," I said, "but why do you push me so far?" I looked around the kitchen in bewilderment. "You don't know when to stop! If I had done something like this, my parents would have *killed* me. Can't you at least act like you're sorry?"

"Mommy," said Harry, tapping harder. I rounded on him.

"Jesus, Harry, what?"

"Rue is eating all the ice cream."

The dog had finished licking the floor and now had the old carton in his paws and his muzzle in its depths.

"I know Rue is eating all the ice cream. I can see that!"

"He's not supposed to eat ice cream, remember? He's allergic."

"Oh, God." I had forgotten. The vet said Rue was getting diarrhea lately because we'd been giving him milk products. "Put him outside."

Harry, oblivious to Byron, ran to do my bidding and Byron looked up from his sobbing, fists clenched. "I hope he eats ice cream to death!" he growled through gritted teeth, glaring at the dog.

"I'm sorry, Byron. But don't take it out on Rue," I said. "You're the one who did something wrong, not Rue."

"Rrrrr," growled Byron, throwing a punch after the dog.

"And I did something wrong, too, Byron. I'm sorry I slapped your face. I'm very sorry, I shouldn't have done that. That was wrong of me. But you were wrong, too. You were very disrespectful. And you and Harry shouldn't have made this mess in here."

"Rrrrr," Byron growled some more, now glaring at Harry as he came back inside.

I gave up. This is what happens when I do something really bad. I get really, really sleepy. Byron growls; I get sleepy. I ordered the children to clean up the kitchen, went and lay down in one of the unused guest rooms, and hoped for the best. Maybe Sean would materialize. I pulled the covers and the brilliantly clean, pure white sheets up over my face, and swooned in a luxury of Clorox and down. I woke up an hour later with Harry and Byron bouncing excitedly next to me. "Guess what, Mommy? Guess what? Guess what?" said Byron. He seemed more recovered from my lapse of sanity than I did.

"Don't bounce on the bed," I said.

"I'll tell her," said Harry. "I saw it first."

"I'll tell her."

 "No, I'll tell her."

"Rue…" began Byron.

Harry interrupted him. "Rue made a mess …"

"I'll tell her," said Byron.

"… all over the front porch!" continued Harry.

"And there are guests coming!" Byron crowed triumphantly.

"I was going to tell her that," said Harry. "I saw them first."

"Poo-poo," crowed Byron.

"Diarrhea," corrected Harry.

I sat up in a panic, pawing at the curtains. "Guests? Who is it?"

Two strangers, a man and a woman, had pulled up near the house and were standing beside their car stretching, looking around furtively. Rue ran up to them, his whole body wiggling and wagging, and immediately stuck his nose between the woman's legs. She jumped.

We did not have the kind of B&B where strangers just stop by. We are hidden away in the woods, and normally only guests with reservations came to the house. Somehow, these folks just found us. But what if I made reservations that I forgot to put into the book, and they were expecting to use the room I had just been sleeping in?

"Jesus Christ Almighty," I said. "Which porch?"

"The *big* porch," said Harry, with meaning. The big porch was the guest entrance. The little porch was ours.

I snapped orders and Harry came to attention. "Get paper towels and cover the poop up. No, no, cover it up with newspaper. Hurry!" Harry ran. "Byron, go outside and distract Rue. Get him to run into the back yard so he doesn't bother the guests." Byron shot-putted off the bed and raced outside in his socks. I ran out onto the little porch.

"Hello," I called, waving.

The man stopped stretching and shaded his eyes, though it was not really sunny. "Is this a B&B?"

I looked at his car in dismay. It was a Jaguar, the expensive car my father always wanted but never got to buy. As a B&B owner, I can state with authority that you do not want expensive people who drive the car your father could never afford showing up on your B&B's doorstep when your children have just had an ice cream riot in the kitchen and the dog has just had an accident on the front porch.

"Yes, it is," I said. "Can I help you? Do you – uh – have a reservation?"

"No," they said, "we just want to take a look."

The man and woman approached. The man was stocky and wore a suit. The woman looked like a model, very tall and skinny, dressed in black leather and tan skin, too beautiful for the rural air. As they came closer, I could see they were both really young. Not even worn around the edges. The woman had heels on, which didn't work well in the gravel, and her smile was so dazzling it could give you a sprain-of-the-neck-other-than-whiplash.

"Is this a Bed and Breakfast?" the woman repeated.

"Yes, it is. We haven't done our landscaping yet, ha, ha," I said. Our landscaping, in addition to our basement renovation, also has been in the planning stages for five years now. In the depths of the woods, our front yard looks pretty much like an ordinary front yard. In fact, the whole house looks pretty much like an ordinary house, which is exactly what it is. "Can I help you?"

"You don't have a front desk?"

"Uh, no," I said. "We're just a B&B, not a hotel."

"Oh," said the young woman, giving a sniff. Then she turned her head toward the front porch and sniffed again, a slight frown on her face. I leaned forward and sniffed, too, and the woman pulled her neck in. I couldn't smell anything except her perfume.

"We'd like to have a look around," said the man, gesturing past me.

"Well," I hesitated. I was about to say that we were full today and you have to call ahead if you want to look around my house, when the lady turned her head toward the front porch with a frown and sniffed again. "Okay, come in," I said quickly.

Immediately, I regretted it. They stepped into our private sitting room, which was stacked with the usual array of papers, books, magazines, toys, shoes, coats, coffee cups, newspapers, more toys, string, tape, dog bones, and other unidentifiable items.

"This is our private space," I said. "Guests don't usually come through here."

"Oh, thank you," said the man. I wasn't sure if he were thanking me for the privilege of walking through our private space, or for the fact that guests usually didn't have to.

We walked through the kitchen. The boys had done a semi-job of cleaning it up. The floor was semi-clean, and the counters were semi-chocolate. All of the ice cream containers were piled on top, leaking over a continent of newspapers. It was terribly embarrassing. As we finally passed on into the living room and dining room, I regained my confidence. The guest quarters were always kept spotless and, on the inside, our house really was very beautiful.

"Where are you from?" I asked them as I showed them the two

unused guest rooms.

"We're from Marginal-dot-com?" said the man. I nodded my head knowingly. Actually, I meant where did they live, but maybe they lived on the job.

"He started the most successful dot-com of the '90s," said the woman. "He turned a profit in his very first year!"

"Wow."

"We're celebrating," said the young man. "It's our tenth anniversary. I'm probably going to rent all the B&Bs around here for a weekend."

"Really," I smiled. The woman ran her finger over the bedside table to see if there was any dust. There wasn't. I noticed she wore no wedding ring. "Gee, you two don't look old enough to be married ten years. Anniversary, huh? Any children?"

They laughed self-consciously, and I was pleased to note a dull glow on the woman's cheek. I figured they'd only just started dating.

"Oh, it's the *company's* anniversary," she said with a trilling laugh, not looking at Mr. Marginal.

We returned to the living room. Outside the wall of glass sliding doors, Harry and Byron were playing tackle with the dog in the back yard. Behind the trees, the setting sun edged the clouds with pink and magenta and molten white; the gloom drifted in through the underbrush, making the three of them look a little like a Vermeer.

"Oh, you have *children* here?" came from Ms. Marginal in a vague and disapproving tone.

"Oh, no," I said. "They're just a couple of Fresh-Air Fund kids." Sean claimed the Fresh Air Fund helped save his life and the organization had a special place in my heart.

Ms. Marginal gave me a startled look, a smile hovering in case I was making a joke.

"Ha, ha," I said.

"Oh," said Ms. Marginal.

"You have a beautiful place," said Mr. Marginal.

"Thank you," I said, opening my reservations book. "What weekend were you interested in?"

They named a date nine weeks hence. I looked it up. I had no reservations for the entire month.

"Oh, I'm so sorry," I said, smiling politely and closing the book. "I'm all booked." After all, I own my own business, too!

As I was escorting them back to their car at a respectful distance, the woman leaned over to the man. "It's better anyway," she murmured in a low voice. I didn't think she intended for me to hear, but she was not trying hard to whisper, either. "Did you see that kitchen? God!"

God at that moment seemed to be listening, because a stiff wind blew up, and suddenly, large pages of the *New York Times* were billowing forth on the rough air. I leaped forward, trying to catch them. One of them whanged right into Ms. Marginal and wrapped itself around her leather butt. It stuck there for a moment, whether held in place by wind or dog poop, I was not sure.

"Oh, I'm so sorry," I said, grabbing the newspaper off of Ms. Marginal's rear. "Somebody left the newspaper on the porch!"

She shrugged and sat down on the cream-colored leather seat of the Jag. There was a whiff of a very bad smell, and I skipped off to the garbage cans with the paper as she peeked sideways under her shoe. Mr. Marginal slid in behind the wheel.

"Drive carefully!" I waved to the disappearing Jaguar. One of the tail lights was out. The Marginals probably did not know how to replace the bulb. Sometimes, that high-end stuff just isn't worth the trouble. Now that I considered it, my father should have been happy with his Subaru wagon. It had been, in many ways, a really superior car.

NINETEEN: A MEAL IS A BATH AND A BATH IS A MEAL
April to September

*T*HE visit from the dot-commers had one positive, albeit painful effect. That Saturday evening, instead of going to the movies as is our usual wont, the four of us spent several grim hours thoroughly cleaning the sitting room and the kitchen, not to mention the porch. I was feeling very sorry for myself and managed to sneak in several isolated visits to the freezer for the chocolate Tofu ersatz ice cream sandwiches that were saved from the children's ravages by virtue of being healthy, and followed that up with one of the jumbo chocolate bars we were supposed to sell for the Little League fund-raiser.

"Why is it we always come last?" I asked Sean as we were sorting through his scientific, music, history, and home-building magazines, trying to find some that he would allow me to throw away.

"What do you mean?" said Sean.

"You know," I said. "Our housecleaning. Our laundry. Our construction jobs. Everything for us comes last."

"Everything we do is for us," said Sean, sitting down at the kitchen table with his nose stuck in an old *Architectural Digest*. "For us and the kids."

It was true in a way, but somehow that answer was not satisfying. I took advantage of Sean's rest period by slipping ten ancient *Scientific Americans* into the recycling bin. "Yeah, but look at the kitchen. We spend so much time in here, and it always gets cleaned last."

"It shouldn't come last," said Sean from behind the magazine. "This kitchen is the first thing we should clean."

"Yeah, you mean *me*, not *we*." The heat began to glow in my neck.

My hair started to prickle. "This kitchen is the first thing *I* should clean, right? You think I should keep the kitchen clean. I'd like it to be clean all the time, too. You always say 'we' when you really mean 'you.' You mean, 'The kitchen is the first thing *you* should clean' but you just don't want to say it because you want to say '*we*,' like you mean…"

"I did not say '*you*,' " Sean interrupted. "I said '*we*' and I meant '*we*.' Okay? Can I read my magazine for a minute please before *we* start working again?"

Sean claimed that I always started a fight with him whenever he sat down to relax, which was completely untrue. Especially in a case like this when he was doing something really annoying. Like sitting down and relaxing. However, I didn't have the opportunity to get into a really good fight with him because suddenly the children, who had sneaked unnoticed from the scene of the crime outside to play in the night, shrieked, then shrieked again.

Sean and I both bolted for the door.

"He's got a possum," shouted Byron, dancing up from the starry darkness into the pool of porch light.

"A possum, a possum," cried Harry, dancing up behind Byron.

"Rue?" I asked. "He caught a possum?" I could see the dog trotting excitedly toward us, head held high, something in his mouth.

"It's *dead*," the children shrieked.

"He killed it?"

"No," explained Harry. "It was *already* dead. He dug it up."

"Oh, no," said Sean, looking sick. "Don't let him eat that. Honey, *do* something."

"How do they know it's a possum?"

"Who cares *what* it is, that foul beast!"

Now, I had no desire to see the dog eat a dead and rotten animal, but more because it seemed remarkably unhealthy to me, plus I anticipated there might be vomit to clean up later on, rather than because the nature of the dead thing revolted me. In fact, I was curious to see it. On the other hand, Sean's revulsion was a shudder of the soul: a terror of the unbearable darkness of not-being, the unraveling of the unbeautiful, and it made me wonder about men. Sometimes they were so squeamish! Blood, dead animals, poop. They had a really hard time with stuff like that. I guessed it was a part of the dog-mind in which women had superiority. Most men had no problem when it came to the growling and the competition and the snarking for position in the pack. But boy, you confronted them with the flattened corpse of a harmless little mouse or a routine dirty diaper, and they ran screaming.

Sean was getting ready to faint. "Get it away from him," he croaked.

"Rue, come here!" I demanded. "Come here, boy."

Rue paid no attention to me. He was engaged in play with his litter-mates. The boys made mad dashes at him. He stretched his hind quarters into the air, his head thrust out close to the ground, tempting them, then whirled off as they rushed him, the prize stiff in his mouth.

"I will never," groaned Sean, "*never* let him lick me again."

The boys stopped running, panting hard, and Rue took the opportunity to lay the desiccated corpse on the ground and roll around in it.

"Mommy," panted Harry, always the logician. "Now I know why he stinks so much sometimes. He likes to roll around in dead things!"

Byron, always the wonderer, said, "Mommy, *why* does he like to roll around in dead things?"

If you thought about it, that was a good question. Why would a dog find odors that are repulsive to humans inviting enough to bathe in? My personal opinion was that dogs did not judge the living and the dead. For a dog, both were equal ingredients in the hasty pudding. A smell was a smell was a smell, and the stronger, the better.

"Well," I said to Byron, trying to answer in a way that was truthful and yet circumspect, so that he did not get the impression that I actually *approved* of rolling around in dead things, "I think he likes it."

Now that the boys had stopped chasing him, I could get Rue's attention. "Rue," I said authoritatively, making a fist and holding it in front of me. "Leave it!" This was a command that we learned at dog-training class, and Rue immediately dropped the corpse from his mouth, though he did poke it with his nose once, just to demonstrate the fact that it still belonged to him. I was delighted that there was someone in the family over whom I had dominion, and I turned a triumphant smile to Sean, who was deeply impressed.

Slowly, I approached the dead creature of the night. In the porch light, I could see its long hideous snout and rows of grimacing teeth attached to a gnarly backbone, a few rags of fur here and there, and a long tail curled into a final wave of goodbye.

"What did it die of, Mommy?" said Byron.

"Old age," I said.

"How do you know?" demanded Harry.

"Because it's not all torn up. If an animal got it, it would be all torn up."

"Maybe a coyote ate its entrails," argued Harry, who preferred a more violent explanation.

"Why do things die of old age, Mommy?" continued Byron.

"Jeeze, Byron," said Harry, contempt dripping from his voice. "Haven't you ever heard of *heaven*? How do you expect to get there if you don't die of old age?"

I was impressed that Harry realized it took an entire lifetime to learn how to be good.

"I don't believe in heaven," said Byron. "I believe in reincarnation."

"We don't believe in reincarnation," said Harry. "Hindus believe in reincarnation. We're Christian."

"Of course there's reincarnation," said Byron, invoking Walt Disney and *The Lion King*. "Everything recycles in the Great Circle of Life."

"Isn't heaven real, Mommy?" Harry demanded.

"Well," I equivocated, trying to think of what Joseph Campbell would say in this situation. "It's kind of a metaphor."

"Yeah, but why do things *get* old?" Byron insisted.

"Because," said Sean, "they have to live long enough to become a burden to their children."

I managed to pick up the possum in a plastic bag, but Rue ran off with the tail. At first I hoped it was just a black stick, but then, as he began to actually chew it up, I had to admit it was probably the tail. It took days before everyone felt the possum cooties had recycled enough to let Rue lick us once more.

That night, Byron had the night terrors again. I was not sure if it was because of the possum and the lick of death, or because I slapped his face in an uncontrollable rage earlier in the day, or just because his particular brain had ionic storms as it recycled the electrons of the living and the dead. I caught him as his little feet were pounding up the stairs.

"Byron," I whispered, scampering up after him. There were guests sleeping upstairs and I didn't want to scare them.

Mute as usual, he turned with blind eyes and ran back down past me, into the kitchen. He whimpered and his face crumpled with terror as he held up a hand, shielding himself from ghosts and visions. Sean came in and together we coaxed him back into bed. He settled down, and I thought he was asleep when he started talking to me.

"I don't like the silence," he said.

"Do you want me to sing to you?"

"The silence sounds weird," he said, looking around, as if he might catch a glimpse of the weirdness.

Was he asleep? Was he awake?

Did it matter?

It worried me sick. Often he seemed perfectly happy, and I thought everything was fine. Then he would have a bout of melancholy and say he was worthless and he wished he'd never been born. And then these night terrors. Was all this illness, or was it a precocious vision into the inconstancy of life?

Coming from my family, how should I know what normal was? I feared Byron would carry self-hatred into his adult life, like my brother. I feared he would develop schizophrenia when he turned seventeen like my niece, Emma. I feared he would become an alcoholic like my father. He already had an alcoholic personality: low self-esteem, fits of rage and frustration, impulsive emotions, and a passion for sugar.

What could I do but try to make him strong now? He had to be stronger than the rest of my family, strong enough to ride out the storms that came his way. I resolved once again to find him a child psychiatrist. I sang to him quietly, a silly song I made up when the boys were babies.

"It doesn't want to get me, you know," he interrupted.

"Something in the dream?" I asked.

"It wants to get everyone!"

"The whole family?" I struggled to understand.

"The whole world. The whole universe. Everyone."

"What is it Byron?" I urged in a whisper. "What is it that wants to get everyone?"

But sleep had taken him. He did not give me the answer.

TWENTY: MY PHILOSOPHY OF LIFE, or,
YOU BETTER BE LAUGHING, TOO
September

*S*EAN was back on the job again. It was September, and the kids were back in school. On Monday, I got up at 5 a.m. to make Sean lunch. Salami and turkey sandwich with lettuce and mayo, sliced tomato on the side, raw vegetables and dip, an apple, water. He liked to buy the stuff he wanted and then get me to surprise him with the day's combination. My friend Denise, an ardent feminist, couldn't understand it.

"You work!" she said. "Why doesn't he make his own lunch?"

"It makes him feel loved," I explained to her. "Feeding him. Don't forget, he didn't have a mother."

I hid a little note under the apple. "Hang in there! Only a few more hours." Union work was hard, especially the first day back on the job. When he came home, he would collapse on the couch, eat dinner, drag himself into his music room, and slowly come back to life as he played his guitar. Then I'd probably get mad at him because he hadn't helped with the dishes. I'd stomp around in the kitchen feeling sorry for myself. Didn't I work? Wasn't I a professional, too? Was I a professional housekeeper, or what? What was I, a professional Mommy? I'd get tired. Exhausted. I'd leave two pots and all of the glasses unwashed, get in bed with the heating pad on my back, call the children and force them to listen while I read *Harry Potter and the Chamber of Secrets* aloud for the third time. By the time Sean got in bed, I would be filled with wizardry and magic. I would have forgotten that I was mad.

O, what would I do when they all grew up and left me?

After the boys went to school, I took a hot shower, scrubbed myself all over with a loofah, drank herb tea with honey. Then I was ready for battle. Fight, fight, fight! That was my motto. Keep trying to find that enemy. Since I'd been considering finding a child psychiatrist for Byron for some time, I already had a good idea whom to consult: my friend Martha, a writer and editor, who had a daughter with a problem.

If I had had a girl, she would have been a lot like Nell, who was nine, only she would have looked like me instead of Martha. Sometimes I fantasized that Nell was my little girl. She was pale, with thick, straw-colored hair, straight as sticks, and a spray of pale freckles over her delicate nose. She was very thin and got sick to her stomach when she was nervous. She was so narrow she could hide in the shadow of a galvanized fence.

Nell loved anything to do with art. Martha was always murmuring, "We're making candles" or "We're tie-dying" when I went over to pick up Tommy, the little flame-headed rocket who was Byron's best friend. I was jealous of Martha and Nell, I had to admit. Imagine being asked to make candles instead of Lego barriers for the toy soldiers to hide behind when they shot each other. *Pow, pkkkkuuuu, kkkkrrrommm!*

Martha was not working that day, and Nell was home with a cold. Nell stood sideways behind her mother at the front door and leaned forward, smiled, so that I saw only one dimension of her: a sliver of hair, an eye and one hand.

A really good child psychiatrist had finally diagnosed Nell's bad stomach. She did not have an ulcer. She had a phobia. Claustrophobia. She was afraid of confinement. Afraid of being trapped. She was afraid to get on the school bus with forty screaming children. She balked at eating in a restaurant. She would not go on a trip to which she could not call a halt. She was afraid of sitting in the center of the center of the theater, where *exit* did not exist.

Nell refined the meaning of the word "alone."   She was and she was not, twisting to a wisp that disappeared into sacred invisibility. To be or not to be was not the question for her, but rather, how to be *and* not be at the same time. The power of her growing self was inside of her, but how could it march forth to bruit herself to the loud and tangible world? She dared not let it out. Her pale slips of fingers ceaselessly shaped *art*. The power caromed off her visible self-control, and it clanked fearfully within. Caromed and clanked, yes. The power was a fearsome thing. It demanded absolute control over one's circumstances. Nell must be able, at any necessary nanosecond, to *escape*. Instinct instructed her. Escape was essential. Else, in a space too confined for the individual spirit, she would be crushed, annihilated.

I understood because I suffered the same thing, but Martha found it difficult to imagine. She consulted with me about *phobia*.

"It is a terrible feeling like you can never explain," I said to her. "As if you are surrounded by shrinkwrap plastic. The world looks like it's in the wrong end of a telescope. Your body parts feel disconnected. Your heart pounds so fast you think you are having a heart attack. You're absolutely convinced that you are about to die." In my mind, I was stumbling out of my parents' house, gasping for breath, my arms and legs shaking, the screaming meemees in my ears, the failing world in my eyes, hurrying down the country lane to nowhere.

"Nobody should have to go through that alone," said Martha.

She gave me the name and number of the psychiatrist who was helping them overcome Nell's phobia. When I got back home and called, I found out I had to wait two weeks for an appointment. I called the pediatrician and he prescribed a sedative to help Byron sleep. That gave me another idea, and I called a sleep disorders clinic and made an appointment for Byron and me to spend the night at their clinic. Should I be tested as well as Byron, I wondered? I was so exhausted all the time. But no, of course, I slept like a stone whenever and wherever. It was not a sleep dis-order; it was the Order of Mommy (somewhat like the Order of the Royal Cross) and here was the order: First children, then husband, then job, then community, then house (except when "community" was coming over, when "house" moved up a notch), then me. Then sleep. Hey, who was complaining? Not me, I had a wonderful life, but the maintenance was a killer.

When I got home, I called Boston family therapists, but all I got was message machines. Then I cleaned the kitchen, corrected student papers, prepped for class, wrote the synopsis for the overdue "Sprains of the Neck Other than Whiplash," answered the B&B e-mail, paid the bills, picked up the kids, went to the grocery store, made dinner. Then it was early evening, and I was driving south to New York City to my class, over the high span of the George Washington Bridge, down into the long necklace of lights moving along the edge of the Hudson River. I was thinking about my brother, how hard it was for him to do the right thing. There was a poem in my mind for Carter, but it kept turning into a song. I heard the music in my head. I pictured him in Central Park with Lyndsey. He had just done something to make her really angry, and she stalked off. He knelt his cumbrous body down to earth and picked a flower from the garden, something tall and blue, like an iris, something to offer apologies and regret.

As I approached downtown, I couldn't help searching for the missing space where the World Trade Center used to be, but I couldn't tell exactly where darkness had replaced the light. It left me with a lonely, achy feeling. In months following 9/11, they sent columns of tall, blue light into the sky to tell us where it was, to ask us to remember. Blue of sad jazz. Blue of the spirit. Blue of the Blue Fairy who helped Pinocchio tell the truth. But for me, the truth for me was a blank.

First, do no harm. If that was a doctor's credo, then we needed a doctor for the world. You would think that would be a savior, like Jesus or Mohammed. Jesus or Mohammed? *Oy vey!* Isn't that how we got into trouble in the first place? Why did there have to be so *many* saviors? Couldn't we just have one?

In the middle of book club, soon after 9/11, my sweet and gentle friend Helena burst out with a rant against religion. Look at all the division it has caused, she said. Look at all the hatred based upon religion. We're better off without religion, she said. Which delighted me in a way, since I'd been feeling guilty for the past year about failing to force the kids to go to Sunday school. It was such an exhausting struggle, not to mention the fact that Sean insists he's a Druid and won't back me up on the steps of the community church where the children balk. Not that I believe in the Christian dogma, but it did seem to me more likely that they'd grow up to be sane and happy and unaddicted if they had a little early-childhood brainwashing. The ABCs of how to love. Somewhere, at that very moment, someone else was teaching children the ABCs of how to hate.

But of course, religion is just the excuse. The parameters, the battle-lines drawn down rifts of heritage. The metaphor for cause. Underneath it all are just the plain old ordinary human failings: lust, rage, intolerance, arrogance, envy, greed, fear. Which could be cured only with the plain old ordinary human virtues: forbearance, patience, humility, courage, love, tolerance, generosity. Oh my God, that sounds dangerously like *religion*! How can you win?

When it comes to terrorism, religion isn't the problem, no more than it is the root of addiction. Religion is just fine. The problem is self-deception. It's the problem with my brother; it's the problem with society. Of all the human failings, self-deception is the worst. Not the most obvious, because it doesn't leave others bereft, like stealing or killing. Nor is it especially painful, because it doesn't wound like cruelty and intolerance and indifference. But it is the most dangerous. The most insidious. The most difficult. It is self-deception that leads us away from the right path into self-righteousness. It is self-deception that enables the religious man to claim he kills in the name of God, self-deception that enables the terrorist to presume he is not drunk on power. It is self-deception that enables the addict to continue to abuse without seeking help. And it is self-deception that leads my brother down the path to his own destruction.

I headed down West Fourth Street, braked to avoid the dope pushers who tentatively congeal like grease gone cold amongst the shadows of Washington Square Park. The park near the university is a traditional hang-out from which the pushers were rousted every few months in a burst of civic frenzy. They japed together, muttered *smoke* to passersby, hooked the occasional student too foolish to hurry on.

But what is more difficult than to be honest with oneself? Self-deception is so easy. It feels so much better. Self-deception can make you into whatever you want. Self-deception comes so naturally, you hardly notice it at all. On the other hand, self-honesty can hurt like the dickens. It can totally wreck the structure upon which your self-esteem is built. Furthermore, to be honest with oneself, one has to discover the truth. And the truth, oh my word, is a slippery thing.

Politicians and public relations experts are well aware of just how slippery truth is, and that is why most of us instinctively hate them so much. They are so good at making "pollution" sound like "on the way to clean water" and "sex" sound like "I never knew that girl" and "war" sound like "the fight against evil." The fight against evil takes place within oneself, thank you very much, and all the rest is boon-doggle.

Or I might say: The fight against evil takes place within oneself, and all the rest is self-defense. Not that I think there's anything wrong with self-defense. I'd shoot a man dead if he tried to kill me or my loved ones. It's just that where does "self-defense" end and "war" begin?

Don't bother me with the truth, says Sean, *I've already made up my mind!* The truth is so slippery, so dependent upon knowing yourself as well as the world, it is easy to slip off into another world, a made-up world, a kind of imaginary world where truth doesn't hurt. A place where I am right and you are wrong. Where I am good and you are bad. Where I am powerful and you are weak. A world where it feels good to be me all the time. Where it feels, in fact, great! Fabulous! Where it feels … well … *high*!

When Joan Didion wrote her famous essay on self-respect, she hit the nail on the head. Failure, disillusionment, *humiliation*, can be the beginning of real self-esteem. Disillusionment gives you the chance to see the truth. When Didion failed to make Phi Beta Kappa despite her high IQ, she was humiliated. She might have chosen to retreat into the certitude of her brainy numbers and breezy attitude, and call those who failed to nominate her fools, but instead, she chose to look at the truth: She had failed to get the grades. How embarrassing and painful. How honest and liberating.

That evening, I stood before my writing class, trying to teach them how to do things with words. *You can't hope to pack everything into one sentence, even one paragraph,* I told them. You have to take your time, let it unwind like a ball of string, slowly, then let the reader gather it all back up again. Language cannot represent reality because it is linear, not three or four dimensional the way a moment of understanding is. Your reader can understand only after listening to the whole thing.

But who listens to the whole thing? When is the moment of understanding? How long does it take to get to the truth? Who is willing to go all the way? Oooo, it makes me shudder! Who wants to look into that pit where me, myself, and I are all vain and self-centered and defensive? It hurts, it hurts, it hurts. It makes me feel like such a ... such a ... vain, selfish, absurd ... *ass!*

What else can you do but laugh out loud? There is just no other way to bear it. Should I feel like the slime I thought I was when my drunken father abused me? Should I feel like the nothing I felt I was when my own *Phi Beta Kappa* mother mocked me? Never! Or rather, never again! I can laugh because I know I am also a good person, and even better, I know that you are just as bad as I am. Well, maybe not "bad," but you aren't perfect, either. Hey, you better be laughing, too!

The truth will set you free, they say, but what if I go through that horrible old prickerbush thicket and slay the dragons and find the holy grail, and it doesn't make me happy in the end? Now that's a twist. What if freedom does not equal happiness?

Personally, I think it does, but it isn't the kind of happiness that is feeling *high*. It is sort of like "mature love." Not falling in love, but the kind of love they talk about in books on relationships, when you've gone through all that divine madness and become disillusioned and stuck together anyway and then you have what's called "mature love." *Ick*, right? Well, it's not the stuff of movie stars, but I'm done with the divine. I'll take ordinary reality any old day. Because sometimes, despite my ambition and my inadequacies, I find a joy stealing up upon me when I am raking the leaves under the beech trees, or when I am kissing my child goodnight, or when my husband and I laugh over the dog's antics, or when my girlfriend and I chatter about important educational and caloric issues, or when I am driving down the road where the fallow fields rise into distant mountains, and I think: How did I get so lucky? And that's all the heaven I need.

TWENTY-ONE: NUMERO UNO, 1999

*T*HEY are not moving the furniture out of the way fast enough for Carter. Mom and I stand by our table, where the hostess has just left us. Another, smaller table and chairs are blocking the way of Carter's scooter. He can't get through, and the hostess did not notice. The young waitress has hurried off as well. Lyndsey has gone to look for somebody to rearrange the furniture. Carter cranes his neck angrily, looking around for someone to help.

"When did he start using that scooter, Mom?" I murmur. Mom and I are visiting Carter and Lyndsey for the weekend, and Mom is taking us out to dinner. We are going to attend Carter and Lyndsey's Summer Solstice celebration the next day. I have not seen Carter in a couple of months. In the morning, I notice, he rolls around in an office chair in the kitchen. Roll to the fridge for milk. Roll back to the cabinet for a bowl. Roll to the other cabinet for cereal. Roll to the drawer for a spoon.

"Not long ago," says Mom, also craning her neck for the waitress.

"Why doesn't he get up? He can get up, can't he?"

"Sure, he can get up."

The scooter is a battery-powered cross between a moped and a tricycle, beige, the color of worn, old-lady shoes. Carter keeps it plugged in by the front steps of the house. Evidently, he goes nowhere without the scooter now. Carter no longer walks the dog. Now, he scooters the dog. He has a "disabled" tag hanging from the rear-view mirror in his car and he parks in the disabled spots. Carter is the first in and the first out. He is numero uno.

He wants to ride the scooter up to the table where he will use it instead of a chair, but the back wheels won't fit between the chairs of two opposite tables. Can't these people in the restaurant see he has a disability?

"I can do it, Carter," I say, pulling the chairs back.

Mom comes over and starts pushing the table.

"Mom," Carter and I exclaim at the same time. "Don't."

"I'll do it, Ma," I say. "Let me do it, now."

Mom doesn't pay any attention. "I can do it. I can do it," she huffs. Mom and I pull the table toward the wall as Lyndsey comes hurrying back with the waitress. Carter turns on the waitress angrily, berating her. "Does my eighty-year-old mother have to move the tables around here?"

The waitress flushes, pulling on the table. "I'm sorry …"

"Carter, it's all right," says Mom.

Carter drives through the chairs like royalty. "It's not all right!"

"I'm not eighty *yet*," mutters Mom. Her birthday is two weeks away.

"What took you so long?" he snaps at Lyndsey.

Lyndsey eyes him angrily. "I couldn't find the waitress."

"I told you to look for the *hostess!*"

For dinner, Carter eats rib-eye steak with mashed potatoes, creamed spinach, a side order of fried onion rings, and hot garlic bread with butter. For dessert, Carter eats chocolate mousse cake with extra whipped cream on top. Lyndsey and Mom and I chat politely as we eat our dinners. We do not look at Carter's food. We do not mention Carter's behavior. When we are ready to go, our waitress, another waiter, and the hostess all pull back chairs and create an aisle for Carter. Majestically, Carter scooters out the door.

TWENTY-TWO: DON'T TELL ME HOW TO TELL YOU WHAT TO DO
September

*C*ARTER was again out of the hospital and back home. He did not have pneumonia. He had something like pneumonia that I didn't really understand, especially when my mother tried to explain it.

"It's, you know, something with the fluid," she said over the phone.

"Uh?" I encouraged. "Fluid?"

"He's got too much fluid."

"Where?"

"In his chest, I guess."

"He has fluid in his chest? In his lungs? That's pneumonia."

"Well, I don't know *where* the fluid is. Maybe it's in his blood. He doesn't have pneumonia, anyway." Mom was much more comfortable discussing the intricacies of Stephen Daedalus' inner monologues than the inner workings of a literal being. Metaphor was her thing. Medical terminology left her cold.

"Is he staying on his diet?"

She had just returned from Carter's house. "Well, I guess you could say that."

I detected a note of irony. "What do you mean? What's he doing?"

"Well, he just eats so *much*." She bubbled with frustration. "He says he's on his diet, and Lyndsey says he's on his diet, but I don't see how you could eat so much on a diet." She sighed. "I don't say anything. Just keep the lip zipped. I can't change anything."

"Maybe you should say something, Ma," I urged.

"Well, maybe I should. But he was just so happy to be home, and back with Lyndsey, and in such a good mood."

"He's got to change, Ma. He's going to die if he doesn't change."

Suddenly, Mom's voice got firm and clear. It dropped into the register of hard fact. There was resolution there, and experience. She'd fought this war before, after all. "I can't change him, CL. You can't change him, and Lyndsey can't change him. Not if he doesn't want to be changed. Only he can change. He's got to want to change and he's got to be willing to do anything to change, and if he doesn't want to, well then he will die from it, and there's nothing we can do, and that's just life."

"I know, I know that's true, Mom," I said. "But I really think that we can help. If we show him our support, if we are honest with him and help him see where he's really at. I think that helps an addict to come to terms with his own addiction, it can help him want to change. Didn't it make a difference when you had that intervention with Pop? I found this therapist in Boston ..."

"CL, I'm sorry," she interrupted me with a loud sigh. "I just don't think I can do an intervention." She sighed again and her voice got teary. "I just can't see that hurt in his eyes. I just can't do it."

I was losing her. I could feel her slipping. She just wouldn't kick butt. Didn't want to make him feel worse. She was too soft. But I couldn't afford to lose her. Carter leaned on her so much; she had to be part of it. If we were going to kick butt, if we were going to get honest, she had to be there.

"Ma," I said, "it's not an intervention. Not an intervention. That's not what I want to do."

I was lying. I did want to do an intervention. Why did Carter go on a million different diets and never get better? Because he wouldn't surrender to someone else's program. He was always doing things his own way, and his way didn't work. I thought he had to go back to OA.

On the other hand, I was thinking to myself, how could I call it an "intervention" if he was already on a diet?

The truth was, I need my mother to be there. I was too scared to do the whole thing on my own. Carter was probably going to get really angry at me. Mom was my protection, my buffer zone. However, I didn't realize all this until much later. At the time, I just got squirmy. I needed Mom. If Mom wouldn't do an intervention, I would call it something else.

"You know, he's already *on* a diet, Ma. Lyndsey already confronted him. He's already trying. I'm just thinking more like, family therapy, you know? I had this B&B guest who was here and she used to be, wow, incredibly obese, and she's really healthy now, and she runs this hospital program in New Jersey to help obese people and she felt sure that family therapy was the way to go with Carter. You know, we'll get together to talk about some issues, like the way he is so isolated. We can talk about having friends, and stuff like that …"

"Well," said Mom, softening.

"And we won't spring it on him," I pushed. "We'll tell him we're going to do it. Hopefully he'll agree to it. I've found this great family therapist in Boston, and he will drive out to Carter's house."

"Well," said Mom, "if he agrees to it, I'm willing to do anything to help."

Once again, I was off. I was psyched. I was ready for battle; I was armed and primed. I was going to do a family-therapy-support-group-kickbutt-addictions-intervention where nobody hurt Carter's feelings.

And I had found the perfect therapist. One of the two who called back. He was a specialist in addictions-interventions, a family therapist, and his philosophy was very love-oriented. He had all the proper credentials, was old enough to have had lots of experience, and he had helped people with compulsive overeating problems before. And he was willing to travel. On the phone, he was a good listener, and when he had something to say, it was pertinent and intelligent. I was thrilled. He gave me a few dates on which he could go to Carter's house for the family meeting.

"But what are we doing, exactly?" I nervously asked Dr. Rausch, who had told me to call him Jim. We were on an extended consulting phone call, which was part of the pre-intervention work and to be billed at only 75 percent the regular hourly rate. "I mean, I guess it's not really an intervention any more because he's already on a diet. You know, he's already trying. And it's not like we can tell him he has to go away to a rehab that day or we'll stop speaking to him. And I think all his junk food is out of the house." I felt dizzy talking about it. My stomach was filled with butterflies.

"There are some things that you need to say to your brother," said Dr. Jim. "If you could talk to him right now, if you could say whatever you wanted to say to him, if you could be completely honest without any negative reaction from him, what would you say?"

That was easy. "I'd say, *'You stupid fucking idiot, why did you let this happen to you?'* "

Since this was obviously not the appropriate, love-oriented, helpful kind of comment I thought Dr. Jim was looking for, I stopped there. But he urged me to go on. "You're angry," he said. "That's okay. Just keep going."

"Okay, I'd say to him, 'You're on a diet but you've tried hundreds of diets. How long is this one going to last? You've tried this and you've tried that, but the one thing you have *never* done is you have *never* let somebody else tell you what to do. You are so stubborn. You can't do it by yourself, Carter! You have to let other people help you. *You have to go to OA*. Now I've proven to you that OA is not just Gray-Sheet Nazis. And even if it were, even those gray-sheet meetings would be preferable to killing yourself with food! This is just not right.' I'd say to him, 'Carter, it is killing me and Mom and the family that you're destroying yourself. My boys are losing their only uncle and Sean is losing his only brother. I know you love Lyndsey and look how you make Lyndsey suffer! A diet of 3000 calories? Come on, give me a break! You have to be willing to give up eating as your big source of pleasure in life. You just have to give it up, like an alcoholic giving up booze. You think there's nothing else in life to enjoy? You really think nothing in life but food will give you happiness? Come on, bullshit, man, bullshit! You have to give it up.' That's what I'd say to him."

I was breathing hard and my heart was pounding, but the butterflies were gone.

"So now you know what you are doing," said Dr. Jim. "That's what this family meeting is about for you. You've got some things that you need to say to your brother."

"But I want to help him," I said. "Is that going to help him?"

"I don't know," said Dr. Jim. "But I think it will help you."

"I don't want to help me," I said. "I want to help him. I want him to go to OA and to get healthy."

"You think that's the solution?"

"Absolutely!"

"Then you have to tell him that," said Dr. Jim. "All you can do is be honest with him."

"What I want to do is kick his butt."

"You can't force him to get better, you know," warned Dr. Jim. "He has to choose it for himself."

I thought of all the times he overate and I never said a thing; I just kept on letting him do it. "Yeah, well I'm gonna kick his butt till he chooses to get better," I told Dr. Jim before we hung up.

I called Lyndsey and discussed the prospective dates for the family meeting.

"Do you think he will agree?"

"I don't know," Lyndsey said. "If you show him that it's coming from love, from concern, I think he will. He's being pretty open right now, but that could turn on a dime."

I hung up and called Carter. My heart was thudding again.

"How you doin?" I asked.

Much better, he said. He is taking massive doses of diuretics. "I have to pee all the time," he laughed. "But I can breathe better."

"I've been thinking about something that I think might be helpful for you." My heart started pounding faster. This was it. I was at the top of a long, shiny, steep slide.

"What's that?" he said. He still sounded cheerful, but wary.

"This is something that's really important to me," I said, instinctively appealing to his desire to help others. He'd much rather help someone else than himself. "This is almost more for me than it is for you. You know it's awful standing by and seeing you get so sick and feeling so helpless about it. I feel terrible. I wish I had tried to do something to help sooner. I know I haven't always been the best sister, but I really love you, Carter."

"I love you too, Cete," he says.

Tears began to leak out of the corners of my eyes. "Well, I know that you are really isolated, except for Lyndsey, and I think that the isolation is really bad for you. I know it is. Maybe that's the real reason that you haven't been able to diet successfully in the past, that, you know, you really have no support system. So maybe the family, maybe we could be a kind of support system for you, is what I'm thinking. I feel that if we have a kind of family meeting, with a, you know, therapist, a family therapist who specializes in addictions and families with addictions, maybe it could help. I mean," I hastened to readjust the focus away from him again, "we could *all* talk about the ways *we* are isolated or have trouble with making friends. We could all talk about the kinds of addictive problems we have. You know I have this problem bingeing on sweets, for example. Maybe making some breakthroughs with the family could help you get more connected with other people, you know? I know this really great therapist in Boston, and he's willing to come to your house and meet with us, and we could all be there."

Carter sounded skeptical. "How can family therapy be a support system for me?" he said. "How often could we meet? I mean, I appreciate the thought but even if we met once a month, how far could we get even in six months? And what are we going to talk about? Are we going to spend the first several meetings just trying to figure out what the agenda is? That's very frustrating."

"No, no, that's not what I have in mind," I said hastily. "That's not it at all. That isn't what I meant at all. We'll meet one time. And then maybe we'll meet again if everybody wants to."

There was a dead silence. Then Carter said slowly, "You're not planning to do an intervention, are you?"

I was pegged. I backpedaled fast. "No, no, not an intervention." I laughed stiffly. "You're already on a diet, Carter. Why would we do an intervention?"

"Because I just know that would really piss me off," he continued.

"No, I don't mean an *intervention* at all, ha, ha."

I didn't mention the fact that I *had* been planning an intervention, as it seemed relatively counter-productive at the moment.

"I'm really talking about more of an opportunity for us all to get together and talk about our mutual problems," I added, "you know, how as a family, addiction has been a problem for us. That we could be a support group, not in therapy, but just on the phone. Just to keep in touch."

"Well," he said, "as long as everybody is talking about their own stuff. I don't want the focus to be me and my problems. Everybody has to talk about their own problems."

I suppressed a flash of irritation. Why *shouldn't* we talk about his problems? He was the only one who was dying here! But I said, "We can talk about whatever you think will be most helpful to you."

"I feel very nervous about a meeting that's set up to 'help' me," said Carter, still suspicious. "I don't want people making suggestions and telling me what to do."

And that, of course, was exactly his problem. He wouldn't let somebody else tell him what to do. But I didn't think about this at the time. I thought about wanting him to agree to the family meeting. Nothing would happen without the family meeting. I thought about making it non-threatening.

"No, no," I said. "Each one of us can just talk about ourselves. We'll talk about our own experiences with addiction and isolation and friends, so that we might be more open with each other, so we can function better as supportive people in your life, and maybe we'd even see some important family patterns."

He sounded skeptical again. "How are you going to keep the others from telling me what to do?"

"Because it's something we'll all agree to ahead of time. I'll set it up with everybody that this is what we're going to do."

"What I would find supportive is for everybody to talk about their problems, about what *their* issues are, not trying to give me advice."

"If that's what you would find supportive, then that's what we'll do, Carter. I'm just trying to help break through your isolation. There's no reason you should be so isolated. You've said yourself the isolation is a problem for you."

Finally, Carter agreed to the family meeting. He even seemed to look forward to it. Lyndsey would be there. Mom agreed to go. Caroline would be there. Even Emma wanted to go; she wanted to help. Sean wanted to be there, but he had to stay home with the kids and go to work.

On the phone, I set up the parameters of our discussion. We were each going to talk about ourselves; we were going to talk about how our lives had been and how we had made friends without giving advice and without telling Carter what to do. Everyone felt comfortable and safe.

Holding my breath, I counted the moments until the Big Day came at last.

TWENTY-THREE: SHRINKWRAP
Late September

*M*OM speeds, so she got there first. She was bright-eyed and bushy-tailed when I got to Carter's house, and I was so tense, I was afraid I was going to develop a migraine. Carter was jolly, and Lyndsey fluttered about making herbal tea. Carter had already lost 40 pounds on his new, 3000 calories-a-day diet, and everybody was ecstatic. He didn't look any different, but you could tell he was very pleased, very optimistic. Mom was charged. "Tell me how to do it again?" she asked excitedly. Carter had planned out an entire diet for her based upon the Systems House plan. "I can't remember how to work the chart."

He instructed her on the subtleties of the diet. Did an intervention still make any sense, I wondered morosely? But we were not doing an *intervention*, I reminded myself. Were we? We were merely coming together to try to improve our family *communication*. Right? I went into the bathroom and sat on the toilet for ten minutes, elbows on my knees, my fingers clutching my scalp. I thought I might throw up.

The therapist, Dr. Jim Rausch, arrived at 12:45. We were supposed to start at 1:00 and Caroline and Emma had not yet arrived. Dr. Jim impressed everybody with his tall and handsome demeanor, firm lines of experience set in his face. He had warm, watchful eyes. Lyndsey took him downstairs to the big song room where we were going to meet. I paced upstairs in the kitchen watching the clock. It was 1:04 and Caroline and Emma were four minutes late. What had happened? Carter laboriously navigated down the stairs, puffing and stopping to rest twice. He had just taken his place in the circle of chairs when Caroline and Emma blew in at 1:08. Terrible traffic, Caroline said. I drew a breath of relief as we joined the others and sat down.

"I have just one request before we start," announced Caroline.

Uh-oh, I thought. *Here we go. Now the fighting begins, before we even get started.*

"I'd just like CL to sit on the side, because I can't see her face when her back is to the window."

I was sitting in front of the large, sliding glass doors that looked out onto the lake. "Oh," I said, moving my chair to the side. "I thought I'd be backlit here and you could all see my halo." That got a good laugh and I relaxed a little.

So here we were, poised on the brink of kicking Carter's butt into OA by sharing our experience, strength, and hope with him, when the handsome and wonderful Dr Jim forgot everything I had already set in place.

"Let's establish some ground rules," said Dr. Jim.

"Carter and I and everybody else already agreed on the ground rules," I grinned nervously. "Everybody's going to talk about his or her own experiences with isolation, making friends, and addictions. No advice." I wanted to get on with it.

Dr. Jim continued around the circle, oblivious to the fact that I had already arranged everything for everyone.

"I just don't want anybody to talk behind each other's backs. If we have something to say, we should just say it," said Lyndsey.

"Nobody can storm out of the room," said Carter.

"We'll be speaking for three hours, so we'd better take a little break every hour," said Dr. Jim.

Emma said she did not wish to add any ground rules.

Now, I thought, *we'll begin.*

"I'd like each person to voice their goals for today," said Dr. Jim.

I bit my lip and crossed my arms. Hadn't I already told Dr. Jim the goal? To kick Carter's butt into OA?

"Better family understanding," said Mom.

"More closeness," said Carter.

"Closeness and communication," said Lyndsey.

"Better communication," said Caroline.

Emma said she did not have any goals.

It was my turn. I covertly glanced at Carter. I pictured him happy and healthy in Overeaters Anonymous, with friends and comrades surrounding him. It *could* happen. My heart pounded; my hands shook. It was the moment of truth. "Better communication," I said, staring at the floor.

Dr. Jim moved on. He asked another question, and then another. I was getting a resentment. As we continued around the circle, Dr. Jim kept skipping Emma, as if she were invisible. I figured Dr. Jim did not know how to talk to a person with schizophrenia. (The answer is: The same way you talk to everybody else.) Did Dr. Jim think *ignoring* Emma was going to make her feel better?

We finished with all the "ground work," and a whole hour had already passed, so we took a break. I spent the time in the bathroom clutching my scalp. I had to get things back on track. When we reassembled, it seemed like nobody knew what to say. Dr. Jim said nothing. There was an uncomfortable silence.

"Okay," I said. "I started this whole thing so I will begin."

I began to talk about the saga of my childhood – the story of family addiction, cruelty, isolation, and making friends – and after about five minutes, Carter broke in angrily.

"I don't want to hear about all this," he said. "I've heard about all this before. I don't want to hear you droning on and on in a monotone about the past. What's going on now? I want to talk about now."

Immediately, I burst into tears. How humiliating! The saga of my tortured past was boring.

"Well," said Dr. Jim, "maybe we could try to focus more on what's going on with us in the present."

That *sonofabitch*, I thought, staring at Dr. Jim with my mouth open. Here I was doing exactly what we all had agreed to do, and he took my screwed-up brother's side against me. What was going on?

"That was really hurtful, Carter," I snapped, still crying.

Carter smiled in a cold, self-satisfied way. "Yeah, well now there is something real going on."

"Real?" I was outraged. "You think I'm only *real* when I'm crying?"

"Well, at least there's some real emotion, now," said Carter, still with the smarmy grin.

I felt like I'd been sucker-punched. Suddenly I remembered why I had stopped being friends with Carter for all those years. I looked at the therapist again. He was impassive.

"That's sick," I said to Carter. "That's sadistic. That's like Pop."

Now Dr. Jim chose to speak. "How was that like your father?" he asked.

"He had to make somebody cry to feel connected."

"I wasn't *trying* to make you cry," said Carter.

"But you feel connected!" I accused him.

Dr. Jim interrupted. "Did anyone else have that experience of your father?" He indicated we should go around the circle again. Each person agreed. That was the way Pop was. Everybody except the therapist knew this. We'd all discussed it a hundred times. Everybody spoke except Emma. Emma said nothing. The therapist skipped over her again.

"Look," I said. "I thought we established this from the beginning. I thought we said each of us was going to talk about our own experiences with isolation and addiction and friendships. That's what I was doing. I thought we agreed that's what we are doing here."

The others shook their heads. "Oh, no," they said, "it would take much too long for everyone to tell their story. We'd have to do that in another meeting. That would take all day."

I couldn't believe it. It was a free-for-all.

"Emma," I said, with a resentful glance toward the therapist. "You haven't really said much. Do you want to say anything?"

Her response was firm and immediate, without hesitation and without fear. "I probably don't have anything useful to say about friends," she said. "I don't have any friends. Well, I guess my Mom is my friend. And all of you. I'm too screwed up to have any friends. And I always hurt people. I used to be a different person. That was before I got sick. But that wasn't really me. Now I'm really more myself. But I can't get close to people because I always hurt people. I don't mean to, but I can't help it."

We all assured her that she had not hurt any of us, but our assurances seemed to roll off her consciousness like beads of water off cold and brittle wax.

Everyone was exhausted. We took another break. When we came

back, Carter was ready to tell us what he had been wanting to say all along. I was waiting for the real story beneath his difficulty making friends and his slow withdrawal from society and his compulsive overeating, but instead he talked about how hurt he was that Mom and I were not planning to spend the night at his house after the therapy session. Mom was planning to go back to Caroline's house. I was planning to drive home. Why didn't we want to stay with him?

Mom and I were flabbergasted. "You never asked," we said simultaneously.

"What do you mean I never asked? I *said* I had all these empty beds and stuff."

"That doesn't mean you *want* us to stay," I told him.

Dr. Jim gave a little lecture on communication. Then my brother and sister jumped all over my mother about how she was the one who didn't communicate. She didn't *listen*, they said. Which was a bunch of hooey; the only time she wouldn't listen is when people were *screaming* at her. Mom sat stoically, nodding gravely, agreeing that she was going to try harder. She was going to be a better listener. And she was going to stay at Carter's house for the night.

I was upset. This was not at all what I had imagined. How was I going to kick butt? I had already missed my chance. I looked at the therapist; I looked at my mother's serious face, the color heightened in her soft, drooping cheeks, the eyes moist behind the glasses. *Nobody should have to sit through this at her age*, I thought. *Come on!*

And then it was over. Three hours' worth. Bitterness consumed me; the whole thing had been worthless. If only we had done everything my way. "We have to meet again," I demanded. "Let's meet again and do what we originally planned."

Everyone else agreed. They all seemed pretty cheerful.

As Caroline got ready to leave, she whispered in my ear, "I'm sorry Carter attacked you like that. That wasn't right." Later, I would ask Caroline about Emma's reaction to the family therapy session.

"Total freakout," Caroline would tell me. Emma felt she had hurt and insulted everyone. She felt the therapist insulted her, too.

"How did he insult you?" Caroline had asked.

"He said that it was a beautiful day."

"Why was that insulting to you?"

"Because," Emma had said, "he can see that I am not beautiful."

Terrific, I thought. Family therapy turned out to be *really* helpful for Emma. Indeed, the therapist had insulted her, not exactly in that way, of course, but even a crazy person knows when she is being ignored.

I saw Dr. Jim to the door and restrained myself from kicking *him* in the butt. My face was sullen; I was depressed. "Try to talk to your brother about what happened," he urged me. I nodded. I wondered why he didn't suggest that during the meeting.

Carter was still sitting downstairs. Mom had gone to her room to collapse. I went back downstairs, and Carter, sitting now by himself, gave me a guilty look. "And Carter pummels his little sister in family therapy." He grinned sheepishly.

"I am feeling pretty hurt, Carter."

"I'm sorry," said Carter, reaching out to me. I let him give me a hug. "I guess I didn't realize how unclear I am. I think I'm telling people something, but maybe I just don't really say it directly."

"Yeah, you don't say it directly."

He seemed thoughtful, cheerful, and relaxed. He had found the meeting helpful.

"Carter," I said impulsively, "I want you to go to OA."

"I know," he said.

And I knew, and he knew, that he was not going to go. We did not discuss it further. There was nothing more to say.

TWENTY-FOUR: THE SECRET OF SPORTS
September to October

I slept for what seemed like forever. Thirteen hours straight. I crawled into bed at Carter's house at 6 p.m., right after we ate dinner, and I slept until 7 the following morning. Mom had already left for home, and I left after a quick cup of coffee.

All the way home, I seethed. I plotted and planned the next family meeting. The next family meeting would go the way I wanted it to go. Not this free-for-all family therapy idiocy. What we really needed, I thought, was an intervention.

The next time it would be less angry, I thought. More sharing. More compassionate. More in control. Each person would describe how he or she dealt with the kinds of problems Carter was having. Imagining it made me feel much calmer. We would talk about solutions, I thought, not about complaints. And we would will really kick Carter's butt into OA. I would schedule it as soon as possible.

Nevertheless, when I got home, I did nothing to schedule another family meeting. Instead, I fell into a deep depression and began to obsess about my career. I made notations in my journal. You can always tell how depressed I am by the number and length of my journal entries. The bad years have very thick journals. How had I failed? Let me count the ways ....

Buck up, I told myself. *Think about Pete Rose. Be more like Pete Rose.* Of course, he did have that terrible compulsive gambling problem. But he was a hitter! He was a fighter. He never let up.

Instead of Pete Rose, the image of my father came to mind: I saw him sitting in the living room gloom, smoking, listening to Mahler, saying, "I guess I'm just not good enough…"

Was that my brother's problem? He felt he just wasn't good enough? He thought he was a loser? I felt like a loser, too. And the thing that really scared me was: What if my boys grew up feeling the same way?

If there was one thing I wanted to give my children, it was the faith that they were winners even when they lost. Learning to lose gracefully was surely one of life's most important lessons. Just because you lost this time doesn't mean you will always lose. Just because you are not the best doesn't mean you are worthless. *I'm just an average player*, said Pete Rose. But brother, did he take his average to the heights.

Nowhere did this lesson present itself more starkly than in sports. Little League, for example. Nowhere was it more clearly evident when you have won and when you have lost. Little League was a great place to learn how to win and lose without losing yourself. Baseball, Sean likes to say, represents all of the values of life in full, and Little League is its training ground. We were not teaching our kids how to become athletes. We were teaching our kids how to win and how to lose.

Of the children who participated in Little League, ours seemed to be the most devastated by personal failure. When Harry struck out, he would throw his bat and helmet into the dugout fence, hide his tears, and tell us he was going to quit. When Byron struck out, he would throw *himself* into the dugout fence, beat the earth, and talk about killing himself. Some of the other little kids didn't even seem to *care* that they had struck out. Was this a genetic thing, or had we already screwed them up?

My friend Carol, a truly great Little League coach with six sons, was the expert at all this and I often observed her closely during our Little League games, trying to learn the Secret of Sports.

Last summer, for example. It was the end of May, a blaze of sunlight over the ball field so fierce, we had to shield our eyes. Carol's son Charlie was pitching the game. Byron was in the outfield, falling asleep. Charlie's older brothers were whiz-kid pitchers, but Charlie was having a hard time. The score was six-six with two outs, and it was the bottom of the fifth inning. Charlie was pitching outside balls, inside balls, balls that rolled over the plate, walking one player after the next.

"Byron," shouted Sean, "look alive!" For a moment, Byron hopefully scanned the outfield, then slouched over his glove again.

Charlie walked his third man and it was bases loaded. Charlie took a long look at the next batter, then wound up and let it fly. It was inside and almost hit the batter. The batter knocked dirt off his cleats with his bat and shot a nervous grin at his dugout, where his teammates were going crazy. They were about to win, and they knew it.

Carol called time out and broached the field to talk to Charlie. Charlie stepped off the mound toward her, shielding his face with his glove. Suddenly I realized that he was crying, his little face working as he tried to hold back the sobs. My heart twisted down to the core; I could hardly watch.

This was a revelation. Carol's kids cried too! I never knew. Usually they were so skillful on the field that they had little occasion to cry. In Charlie, I saw the same effort, the same rage and humiliation as my boys experienced, the same ambition to be something he was not. He shielded his crumpled face with his mitt, so that the others might not see his tears. I wanted to rush up and fold him into my arms, to hug him and tell him what a great kid he was. Anything to take away the pain.

Carol knelt and spoke to him. What did she say? I wished I knew. Even when she spoke like that to my own kids, spoke her special, magic sports-words as she knelt before them and looked them in the eyes and told them how to live life and kick butt, I never knew what it was she said. Charlie nodded, then nodded again. He wiped his nose and went back to the mound. He threw another ball, outside. Then he threw three strikes in a row. The inning was over with delirious cheers and praise. Charlie was grinning, and you want to tell me that wasn't a lesson in life worth learning? The Secret of Sports was to take the pain away by yourself. You have to persist. You have to believe. You have to walk through the pain and face it down.

Nevertheless, it is difficult to walk though the pain when you don't know exactly where it's coming from. I was depressed, and I didn't really know why. A few days after coming home from our family meeting, when we were at the Fifth Grade Choral Concert, I was further depressed by this year's crop of kids: So many fat ten- and eleven-year-old girls, as bloated as inner-tubes, galumphing up to the stage in overly-tight dresses and high heels, spangly skirts slit up the thighs, bare bulging midriffs, drooping waistbands and plunging necklines, tanktops stretched skintight over lumpy, immature breasts. What was the ambition of these girls, I wondered, and what would they count as success? Much too little, I was afraid. Was there no one coaching these girls on how to think big? Could it possibly be that our school failed to inspire these girls? The only big thing here was their incipient sexuality, and the passive glance of an overstuffed culture.

I wanted to shout it out in the middle of the hot and sticky school gym: *Hey, this is important, folks.* Stop eating this way! Go on a diet. This isn't cute; this isn't trivial; we have a killer here, a killer stalking our kids! Fat. Yes, and indolence, too. And a failure of ambition.

Where was the good old American know-how? Where was the good old-fashioned work ethic? Where was the pride and the optimism and the knowledge that anybody who tried hard could make it? These girls should have been playing baseball and amazing their parents with math, not slinking around in tight dresses, eating themselves into oblivion.

Feeling you are "not good enough" is hardly the only danger in our society. Not wanting to be better is a danger, too. Losing, after all, can only happen if you are trying to win. Learning how to fail can happen only when you are trying to succeed. Giving up can happen only if you've made an effort. What about the people who don't even try? Who don't dream? People who don't even have a "dream deferred"? Do they implode? Suck society into a black hole?

At least I could say of my brother that he had a dream. He had a dream, but it was the wrong dream. He thought he was trying to build a new society, but really, he was just trying to rearrange those terrible thorns of love so they would not hurt him so much. Carter's true dream was to escape from pain. I guess my father never took him to those places where he could learn to walk through it and get to the good stuff on the other side.

After the school concert, I realized that I was depressed because all my efforts to save Carter had failed. *Didn't quite kick butt, there, did you, CL. Seemed to get kicked around a bit yourself there, didn't you.* How the heck did that happen? Somewhere along the line, I backed off. I lied. I wasn't honest with my mother. I wasn't honest with Carter, either. I wanted to do an intervention, and I let it fizzle. Once again, I got fearful.

I decided I mustn't give up. We would have another meeting, I thought. Or maybe I'd just go by myself again. I plotted and planned dates. Next time, I thought, I'd be braver. I'd really kick his butt into OA.

Then something amazing happened. Carter started to win.

TWENTY-FIVE: SUCCESS
October

*M*Y brother was reading *Sierra* magazine in the bathroom. *Wilderness Rafting Trip,* it said on page 28. The picture caught Carter's eye. It was a group of men and women in a large rubber boat on a swirling river overhung with trees. The front of the boat was kicked up with river spray, and all of the people in the front were holding onto the sides, laughing, wet with foam, while the people in the back of the boat were digging hard into the rapids with their paddles.

Carter remembered the Adirondacks, the heavy fir trees and the pines, the rushing white water. He waded into the river with his waist-high boots, cast his fly line back and forth, back and forth in a large S above his head until the line was played out and the fly landed gently in the quiet eddy beside the rocks.

"Contest" said the heading above the picture. *Can you answer the questions?* The Wilderness Rafting Trip was a prize for winning the contest. If you answered the questions correctly, if you were chosen, you got to go on the trip.

In his mind, Carter answered the questions with mounting excitement. *What is the name of Rachel Carson's famous book? Who began our system of National Parks?* He scanned through all twenty questions. He knew the answer to every one.

Carter decided to enter the contest. An eerie premonition came over him, as if the *Sierra* magazine were telling him something, as if the very wilderness itself were calling to him. He was going to go on that wilderness rafting trip. He was going to get well. He had been chosen.

*   *   *

"I've already lost fifty pounds since June," Carter told me on the phone. "I'm feeling great. Much better." His Systems House diet of 3000 calories was actually working. He told me about the *Sierra Magazine* contest. "I entered this contest, and I just feel that I'm going to win."

My jaw dropped over the receiver. "Wilderness rafting?" I repeated stupidly. "You're going wilderness rafting?"

"Yeah," he said, laughing with delight. "Lyndsey was horrified by the idea. And I have to admit, if I were really honest about my condition, they wouldn't let me go."

He calculated that at his present rate of weight loss, even counting some weeks with zero losses, he could get down to around 275 by next June. "If I can get down to 275, I won't need the oxygen at night. I'll be able to sleep without it."

My excitement mounted. Carter had a goal – a real goal. To get down to 275 and go on a rafting trip in the wilderness. Finally, Carter had made a *commitment* to health.

"Wow," I said. "Carter, that would be really super!"

"Lyndsey is worried about me not being near a hospital if I get a heart attack," he said. "But you can't just stop living because you might die."

"Well," I said, "if you don't win the contest, you can still come visit me next summer and go canoeing or something."

"Even if I don't win the contest," he said, "I'm going to take the trip."

*   *   *

Carter did not have to wait to take his journey. He had already begun.

"I've lost another ten pounds," he told me. I did not have to see him to feel his radiance. Outside my kitchen window, the leaves showed the first streaks of red and gold, and I could glimpse the sun's last light behind the trees.

"So are you still planning to win that contest?"

He laughs. "Yeah, I figure I may not win that contest, so I've been looking on the Internet for wilderness rafting trips for me and Lyndsey.

Idaho looks really good. Colorado is good too, and there's something in New Mexico, but I've never been to Idaho."

"Jeeze, I never knew Idaho had wilderness rafting."

"It's got everything – forests, rivers, wild places. It's a beautiful state."

"I never knew."

"Yeah. There's so much still left to see."

Idaho called to Carter. He spoke to the wilderness-rafting tour guide on the telephone. "So what do you do if somebody has a bad accident or gets sick on one of your trips?" Carter asked casually.

"Well, we've got the first aid kit," said the guide. "And a variety of medicines. And if there is a serious accident – which, by the way, has never happened so far – we are always in touch with our base and they can be evacuated right away."

"Sounds good," said Carter.

"See," he told Lyndsey later, "they can evacuate me right away if anything goes wrong."

Lyndsey rolled her eyes.

My mind was filled with visions of Carter skimming through foamy, roiling rivers and eating gargantuan potatoes cooked in buried coals deep in the forests of Idaho, when Mom called with more good news.

"Well, Carter and Lyndsey are going on a bicycle trip in Maine," she trilled gaily.

"I thought they were going wilderness rafting next summer."

"Well, I don't know, but they're leaving this Friday. Isn't that great?"

"Wow." Now I was picturing gargantuan lobsters and clams baking on a misty, seaside shore. I was beginning to get jealous. I hadn't been on a vacation in years. "How's he going to ride a bike?"

Mom didn't have an answer, so I called Carter.

"I lost another three pounds," he told me proudly. "We're going to take a bike trip in Maine."

I was elated. He must be feeling really good. "Maine," I said enviously. "Wow. So you're riding your bike again?"

"A little. This trip will get me jump-started."

"Are you sure you can ..." I hated to say it, but how could he possibly cycle miles and miles?

Carter knew what I was thinking. "Oh, they have a van that goes along with the bikers, so I can ride in the van whenever I want to. Don't worry."

I could hear him grinning at me.

"Not only that. We're thinking about maybe going to Killington to ski in February."

"Skiing? Vermont?" It was too much for me. "I haven't been on a vacation in *years*!"

"So come with us."

I tried to think of a credit card I had not yet maxed out. I couldn't think of one off hand, but there were always those great Christmas low-interest balance-transfer new credit card offers. "Okay."

"Great. Come biking with us to Maine if you want."

The thought of Sean and the kids stumbling thought a week of B&B chores at the height of the season made me shudder. "Naw." I was happy just to hear him getting better, finally. And I felt a little proud, too. I had helped. Our intervention had worked. "Just go and have a wonderful time."

*   *   *

It was the third day of the trip, and as they reached the top of a hill, Carter drew a sharp breath. "Stop!" he shouted, and the van driver, Ray, braked abruptly.

Carter got out of the van, turning around 360 degrees. Everywhere he could see was color: the rolling yellow and rust hills, the dark green pines, the red and orange maples. The sky fairly crackled with blue, with only a few white clouds floating high above, and the air had a lingering sweetness mixed with the sharp scent of loam, as if flowers were hidden nearby under the fallen leaves.

On the country road ahead, down the long hill and into the woods beyond, rode Carter's bike tour group. They were strung out in a long line. The last in the group was disappearing into the woods below. Carter couldn't tell who it was. Probably Mr. Moskowitz, who was 67 and very careful. In front of him would be Mrs. Moskowitz, giving her husband an endless stream of advice, and then would come the others and way out in front, there would be those two sisters in their black stretch jumpsuits, Franny and Julia Something, pedaling like mad. Carter didn't like hanging out with the group after dinner, making small talk and such, but right now, when he thought about their efforts to befriend him, an immense love and gratitude surged into his heart. How could life get any better than this?

From behind, with a noiseless *whisk* of air, the driver lifted Carter's bicycle from the bike rack and wheeled it up beside Carter. "You want to ride down?" By the third day, Ray was getting to know Carter's routine.

Carter grinned, buckling his helmet. "Thanks, Ray. Time to get my exercise." His left foot rested on the firm, familiar feel of the pedal. He pushed off. For a moment, the bike glided and he rested there, feeling weightless. Then, swinging his right leg over the seat and down, he engaged the pedals in the pump and push against gravity. Ray crossed his arms and watched Carter's great bulk settle gracefully into place.

After three short pushes of the pedal, Carter glided over the lip of the hill. His bike gathered speed until he was racing, the wind in his eyes and on his face, the red and the gold a blur on the sides of the empty road. Faster and faster flew Carter's bike, in one long, spine-tingling rush. The cold brought tears into his eyes, his eyes almost closing against the sun and sharp air, and the tears whipped back from his face. He did not slow down, nor did he brake. He was not afraid. Let the road take him as far as it would.

TWENTY-SIX: GRIT YOUR TEETH
November to December

*I*T started a few days later with a minor cough that wouldn't go away. He coughed and coughed, a deep, twisting rasp in his chest. The cough got worse. One night, when Carter lay down to go to sleep, he could not stop coughing; he was short of breath, even with the oxygen. He spent the night sitting up in his big TV chair. The next day, Carter went to his regular, primary care doctor. The doctor said he had bronchitis and sent him home with an antibiotic and a narcotic cough medicine.

Then the swelling began. First it was in his legs. He went back to the doctor, and the doctor gave him a diuretic. The swelling was edema, which meant he had too much water in his tissues. Why did he have edema? Was it related to the narcotic cough medicine? Was it related to bronchitis? Nobody knew. Carter went home with the diuretic and continued to swell: his legs, his abdomen, finally his testicles. He was coughing and blowing up like a balloon.

"This is scary, Carter," said Lyndsey. "You better call the doctor again."

Carter called his doctor. "Go to the emergency room in the hospital," his primary care physician told him. In the emergency room, other doctors examined Carter. He coughed for them; he showed them the swelling.

"You should call your primary care physician," said the emergency room doctors. They were ready to send him home again.

Then Carter got angry. Doctors really hated it when Carter got angry. He could be incredibly obnoxious. "Something is wrong with me,"

Carter insisted. "You have to figure out what it is. I'm not going back home again."

Finally they took an X-ray of his lungs. He had fluid in his lungs. Fluid was pooling in his body everywhere. They put him into the Intensive Care Unit on massive doses of diuretics.

The first breath of this new crisis came to Sean and me after the early November wind had given the trees their final shakedown, and the air was sharp with wood-smoke and the promise of snow. Byron had taught Rue to roll over, and he needed to tell Uncle Carter about it immediately. He left a message on Uncle Carter's machine, but Uncle Carter did not call back. There was foreboding. Byron whined. Why didn't Uncle Carter call back?

Finally, there was a message on our machine. Carter said he had been in the hospital, but just overnight. He was already back home and he was okay.

The voice in my head whispered, *You'd better call him right away,* but I didn't want to know about it. It was nothing. Carter had said so. Two nights later, Mom called me. Carter was back in the hospital again. Intensive Care.

The world stopped.

"But it's not his heart," Mom said cheerfully. We were relieved that it was not his heart. "He's retaining fluid. They have to keep him in the hospital for about three weeks while they get the fluid out of him."

"Why is he retaining all this fluid?" I asked. She did not know.

I called Carter, and he called me back from the hospital. He explained what had happened, about the coughing and the fluid and the swelling. They had put a tube into his abdominal cavity like a gasoline hose and they were draining off the fluid. It had something to do with this heart not being strong enough to pump the fluid around properly.

Carter was laughing. "I shouldn't tell my sister this," he said. "You know, I'm on all these diuretics, so I have to pee all the time. But my scrotum is so swollen, my penis is just buried. I mean, they're bigger than grapefruits. It's just totally buried. They give me this piss pot that's shaped like a hat; it's called a 'hat,' and I'm supposed to pee into the hat. So I try to pee into the hat but my penis is so buried, it's like a busted garden hose. The pee just goes spraying all around the room."

I giggled and Carter giggled, until finally, we were both laughing hysterically. Carter began to cough and cough. I stopped laughing. I would not tell Mom that it was related to his heart. After all, what was the point?

*   *   *

Two days later, Carter was not so cheerful. He was vomiting into a bed pan. The remains of his breakfast were long gone, and little more than bitter foam came up.

"I want to speak to the doctor," he told the Head Nurse again.

"I told you, Mr. Watson, the doctor will be here at noon. That's when he has rounds. You can talk to him then."

"I need something for the nausea."

"We already gave you something for the nausea. The diuretic is making you nauseous."

"Reduce the amount of the diuretic, then." Carter heaved again.

"This is the amount the doctor prescribed, Mr. Watson. I know you're feeling terrible, but you just have to grit your teeth and bear it. The diuretic is what is going to make you better."

Gritting teeth and bearing it was definitely not Carter's strong suit. We Watsons were fixers. We Watsons were not teeth-gritters.

"Call the doctor," insisted Carter. "Tell him I have to speak to him."

Half an hour later, the doctor showed up. Carter had a long discussion with him about the medications and the stress on his heart. The doctor reduced the flow of the diuretic and gave Carter another shot to quell the nausea.

"Hmmph," said the Head Nurse.

*   *   *

In the hospital, Caroline and Carter were having a wonderful, brother-to-sister conversation. Carter was sitting up, feeling much better.

"They are going to keep me here until they can get rid of the fluid. They think I may be carrying 50 pounds of fluid," Carter told her.

"Fifty pounds?"

"Yeah, you know, I haven't lost that much on my diet this month, but now I realize that's because of the fluid."

Caroline looked at Carter. Even though he'd lost sixty pounds, he didn't look very different. He still weighed around 340. "Fifty more pounds will give you a huge boost."

Carter's round face glowed with excitement; his cheeks were flushed and his eyes were happy. "And then all I need to do is lose a hundred pounds and I'll be back to 200. I haven't weighed 200 since I was in the Peace Corps. Once I get my weight down, I'll be able to do all kinds of things again. I think I'll still be able to go skiing in Killington this February. Maybe we can all go."

Caroline called me from the hospital. Optimism scintillated through the wires. "He was talking about doing all sorts of things," she told me excitedly. "He wants to teach Harry and Byron fly fishing next summer. He's got it all planned out – the diet, how long it's going to take him to lose the hundred pounds. I have never heard him sound so good."

*   *   *

The next day, Mom visited Carter in the hospital. Mom could hear Carter's voice as soon as she got up to the Nurses' Station. She sat down in the little waiting room instead of going into his room.

"What are you trying to do, *kill me?*"

The Head Nurse came striding out of Carter's room, her face tight and grim. It looked like she was gritting her teeth. She snatched up a clip board at the Nurse's Station and went back into his room. Carter started yelling again. He was angry that the nurses woke him up all night to give him medications. He wanted the nurses to let him sleep. How could he possibly recover without any sleep? He'd been awake all night. Didn't they know he had sleep apnea? How was he supposed to get any rest?

Later, Mom called me at home. "Carter yelled at the nurse terribly. He said awful things to her. But she went back in there and listened to everything he had to say." Mom was very impressed with the nurse's courage.

"And you know, when Carter gets going, he can say a lot! The nurse stayed in his room for at least 40 minutes talking to him about what he wanted," said Mom. "She didn't know who I was, because when she came back to the nurses' station, I could hear her talking about him."

Mom imitated the Head Nurse. She sounded like a cross between Clint Eastwood and Julia Childs. " 'Well, that was the most *challenging* patient I've ever had in all my years of nursing. But I knew I could do it!' "

Mom and I laughed. We understood what it was like to deal with Carter when he was angry. We admired the nurse's grit.

*   *   *

Caroline called me later, crushed. "They've transferred him to the pulmonary rehab. He's talking about leaving the hospital altogether."

"But what about the fluid?" I said. "What about the 50 pounds?"

"He can only stay five days anyway," said Caroline bitterly. "Because of the insurance."

*   *   *

Carter did not leave the hospital after five days. He developed an infection in his leg where it was swollen. His thigh became inflamed and dark red streaks spread down below his knee. This was more dangerous than the fluid around his lungs. The doctor didn't know what it was. Phlebitis? Cellulitus? Carter thought it was staph, which he had in the Peace Corps. Mom was scared. "Flea-Bitus?" she asked. "Where did he get this infection from?"

"It's possible he got it from the hospital itself, Mom," I told her uncomfortably. "That happens sometimes – it's called nosocomial infection."

The IV antibiotics were not working; the infection was spreading. He'd die of blood poisoning if they didn't stop it.

It was 7 a.m. on a Wednesday, and I told the boys Uncle Carter was very sick and they were not going to school. We were going to drive up to Boston to see Carter in the hospital and drive back home in one day. I was afraid Carter was going to die and we wouldn't get to see him. If we sped and didn't stop much, it would only take us about five hours each way.

"Come on," I screamed at the kids. I was on edge. They were fighting over which bag of leftover Halloween candy belonged to whom, and I was in a hurry. I grabbed both bags and flung them together. "Just bring it all."

The phone rang. It was Carter. "You better not come." He sounded faint, far away.

"Why?"

"I don't want to see anybody right now. Come later."

What was I going to say? There might be no later?

"You don't have to talk or anything, Carter. I just want to see you."

"I have to sleep," he told me. "I'll be okay. Just come later."

We unloaded the car. Sean went to work and I collapsed on the sofa, exhausted.

"Do we have to go to school now?" Harry asked tremulously.

"Uncle Carter is still sick," mentioned Byron.

I pulled the wooly throw over my head. "Be really quiet," I warned them, "or I might have to take you to school."

They played like perfect angels for the rest of the day.

*   *   *

Finally, the antibiotics worked. Carter stayed in the hospital for three more weeks, slowly improving. We talked on the phone regularly, and I sent him a lot of books and magazines. I thought he must be going nuts from boredom, but for the first two weeks, he felt too ill to be bored.

It was almost Thanksgiving before Carter could leave the hospital. He left me a message on my answering machine as soon as he got home. *Let's not do presents for Christmas this year*, he said. Carter always worried about giving the right presents, about giving enough presents. He and Lyndsey had no money; they were stripped down to the bone on Carter's social security with the medical bills and debt and Lyndsey's struggling income, and anyway, who needed presents? I agreed. My house was cluttered with stuff; I wanted nothing but my family's health.

But when I returned Carter's call, he had been throwing up. He kept laughing as he talked to me, and suddenly I realized, with the taste of panic like tin on my tongue, that each time he laughed, he laughed because he was not crying.

"I can't eat," he said. "I made myself a turkey, just to eat the plain meat, but I threw it all up." He lay on the couch all day, too nauseous to move. "I can't even drink my raspberry soda. Not even raspberry-flavored water. I just throw it all up."

"What is it? Why are you sick to your stomach?"

Now they thought perhaps it was his pancreas. Pancreatitus. Or it was his thyroid. It also might be the new thyroid medication, which they had to increase slowly and so far it was not helping. Or it might be his metabolism.

"All I can keep down is rice and cooked vegetables."

"Oh, my God," I said. "You're on a real diet!"

He laughed. "Yeah, I'm only eating about 1,000 calories a day, but I'm not losing any weight, I guess because of the fluid retention. My thyroid is super non-functional. I'm putting salt on stuff, and I'm not supposed to, but I can't stand it without the salt." He laughed at himself again.

"You are giving up your addictions one by one."

"Yeah," laughed Carter. "I'm being forced to."

"It sounds like you're on a Vietnamese prison diet. You didn't go to Vietnam, and now you're paying for it."

"Yeah, or maybe I'm just being forced to eat like so many people in the world. That's all they have to eat."

"Mmmm." I didn't want a lecture.

"I was doing pretty well there for a while. I was even doing the water aerobics till I got sick again. I thought maybe I would get better, but I guess not."

I hung up and cried. I berated myself. Why did he choose to get better after it was too late? Why hadn't I done family therapy or an intervention *years* ago?

*   *   *

We were not sure whether Carter would be in the hospital or out on Thanksgiving Day. We thought he might be coming to Caroline's for dinner.

"When's Uncle Carter and Aunt Lyndsey coming?" whined Byron, poking his turkey.

"Pretty soon," said Mom.

"They said they might come after we eat," said Caroline, bringing in the salad. It was hard to muster our Thanksgiving feast in her small apartment kitchen, but she was doing an admirable job. I took a second helping of sweet potatoes with marshmallows and prayed Carter and Lyndsey would arrive after dessert. How could we possibly stand by and watch Carter eat? Emma produced her famous homemade pecan pies, and, to everyone's relief, Carter and Lyndsey don't show up until we'd cleared all the dishes. Carter looked pretty much the same, despite his weight loss and his constant hospitalizations. He was very jolly, and he gave Byron and Harry each a ride around the entire floor of Caroline's apartment building on his scooter.

That evening, we played our first and oldest family game, charades. Each of us acted out a title while the others tried to guess. The person with the fastest time won. Carter always played like Dad used to: fast and serious, trying to win. Mom usually lost, but made everyone laugh. That night, for example, Harry guessed Carter's *The Lion King* in seven seconds flat. Mom, on the other hand, began with flowing motions, like a river.

"*A River Runs Through It*," I shouted.

She looked exasperated and began again, this time with big round circling motions with her arms.

"The sun?"

She shook her head vigorously, no.

"Breast exercises?" I remembered my own adolescent efforts to enlarge my flat chest. "Does it have something to do with breast exercises?" Mom started laughing and crossed her legs so she wouldn't pee. Then she started hopping around with her hands next to her ears and Carter laughed so hard I was afraid he'd fall off his scooter. Nobody had the faintest idea what she was trying to say. Finally, Mom gave up, wiping her eyes. "I got to go to the bathroom," she said, "so you better guess now."

"*The Sun Also Rises*," I ventured.

Mom was indignant. "Where do you find a rabbit in *The Sun Also Rises*?"

"But what was this?" I imitated the circling of her arms like a big sun. "That's the sun."

"I told you that wasn't the *sun*. That was supposed to mean *the whole thing*. I was acting out *the whole thing*." Mom always liked to look at the big picture.

"*Alice in Wonderland!*" guessed Caroline.

"Yes!" said Mom, clapping her hands. Her time was seven minutes and twenty-five seconds. Carter was the fastest, but Mom really won the game, I thought, because she made us laugh the most.

It was a happy day for us. As Lyndsey and Carter got ready to go home, I hugged Carter's big neck across the handlebars of his scooter. I thought about the times he rode me on the hard rim of his bike when I was little. It was good to laugh with him at Thanksgiving. *Goodbye, goodbye. This is the memory I will keep of you.*

*   *   *

By early December, Carter was in the hospital again. His body was filling with fluid. He was throwing up. It was not his heart. It was not his liver. It was not his kidneys. They didn't know what it was. Finally, they put a tube into his body and simply drained water off into a bottle, liter after liter. Lyndsey called me one night a few days later, sobbing. "I don't think he's going to make it," she said. "I think this is it." He was in the ICU. His blood pressure was down to 30. All his organs were failing; everything was going.

I was ready to jump into the car and drive to Boston, but before I could make arrangements to go, I got another call. He was stabilizing. He was out of danger.

Two weeks before Christmas, I called Carter in the hospital. It was a good time to talk to him, in the early evening. Sean had taken the kids off to a movie. It was quiet. Carter was alone, too; the doctors and nurses were not bothering him. We chatted for a long time. I told him all about our latest adventures in life. I was not sure if this was the last time I would ever speak to him, or if he would get better.

"Carter," I told him, "I've written a song for you."

I had never written songs before, but I took a lyric writing class and in it, I wrote a song about Carter. I was going to give the song to him as a gift, but now I was not sure Carter would last until Christmas.

"A song for me?" Carter was amazed.

"It's about you. Actually, it's in your voice. I was going to give it to you for Christmas."

"I want to hear it!" he demanded.

"I'm not sure you will want to hear it," I warned him. "It's a sad song. It's a song of goodbye. Are you sure you want to hear it?"

"Of course. A song about me?" he said excitedly. "Hey, I've got an ego! Sing it for me."

"On the phone? Right now?" I was a little flustered.

"Yeah, sing it for me now!"

I switched phones and went into Sean's music room, where I had a tape of the accompaniment.

"In my mind, this song is part of a larger show," I explained to Carter before I began. There was a man and a woman in a park, near a garden of flowers, having an argument. The man was very big and rode a scooter, because he could no longer walk very well. They argued and the woman walked off angrily. The man got off the scooter, went heavily onto one knee, and picked a flower. A boy ran by, and the boy said, "Hey, Mister. You're not supposed to pick the flowers."

And the man said, "Oh, I don't think anybody will mind."

And the boy said, "Flowers are for girls, anyway," and he ran off.

Then the man turned after the woman, as if he were about to go after her, and sang:

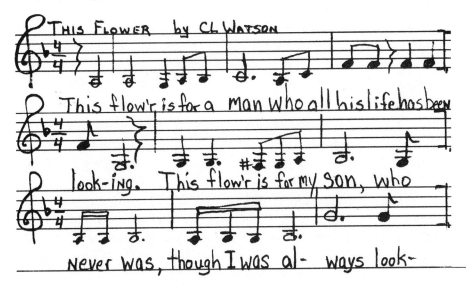

206

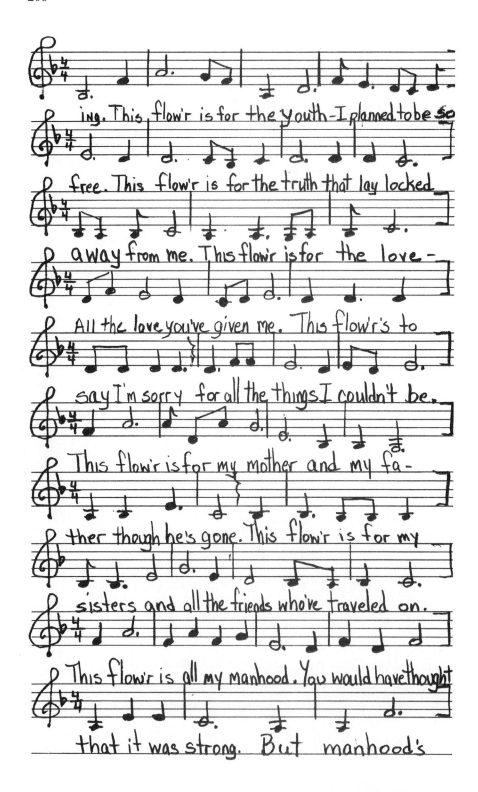

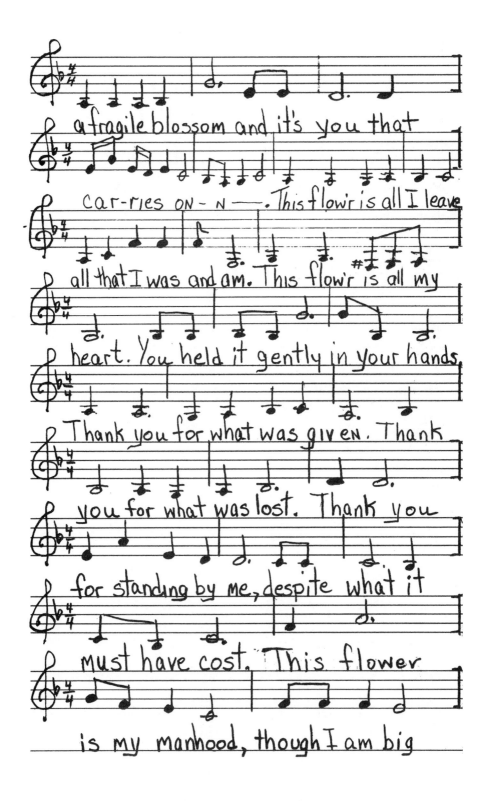

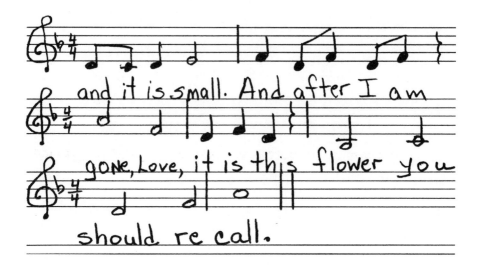

should re call.

At the end of the song, I was crying and so was Carter.

"That's beautiful, CL," he said. "Thank you."

"Well, that's how I feel about you, Carter."

"It says how I really feel," he told me. "I want you to sing that for me at my memorial service."

"Yes," I promised him. "I will."

TWENTY-SEVEN: SPIRITS BEHIND ME, SPIRITS BEFORE
December

*I*T was late afternoon, and Carter was watching the TV in his big chair in the living room with his raspberry seltzer and his telephone and his sleep apnea machine. Lyndsey was getting ready to go downstairs. She was expecting her class to arrive soon. They would shut the double doors to the song room and let their voices go.

"Hon," Carter said, "leave your cell phone on in the song room, okay?"

"What?" said Lyndsey, startled. "I can't leave the cell phone on in there. It will interrupt the class."

"You know, in case I have an emergency." Carter yawned. He always yawned when he was embarrassed.

A terrible rage rose in Lyndsey, making her blood pound in her throat and her ears burn. "No! I can't do that."

"It's just in case."

"I can't do that." She felt like she was suffocating.

"Well, what am I going to do if I have an emergency?"

"Call 911," Lyndsey snapped, running down the stairs and setting the tea pot up in the song room with trembling hands. Before everyone came, she went into the bathroom and blotted her eyes with toilet paper, taking slow, deep breaths. Then she turned on her cell phone.

*   *   *

They were doing more tests in the hospital.

"What I am most afraid of," Carter told Lyndsey, "is that I will be in pain and I won't be able to tell anyone."

"That's not going to happen to you."

"Don't let them do that to me."

"I won't; that's not going to happen you."

"It's my greatest fear in life. Not being able to communicate how I feel."

They gave Carter anesthesia for the procedure. Normally they didn't use anesthesia, but Carter insisted. When it was over, he lay unconscious in the ICU, breathing with a respirator down his throat. He looked terrible. Lyndsey rubbed her eyes. She was exhausted.

"You can go home," the nurse told her.

She looked longingly at the door. "I shouldn't leave him alone."

"I'll call you if there is any change."

"I'll only be twenty minutes away," said Lyndsey. She was staying nearby at her mother's house.

"Go ahead, get some rest," the nurse urged.

Lyndsey went, guilt and relief flooding her drained senses. When she returned the next morning, they were just getting Carter off the ventilator. He was waking up and he seemed to be in pain. He was agitated and sort of choking, and he was motioning to Lyndsey. It was just what he begged Lyndsey to save him from. He was in pain and he couldn't communicate.

"What are you doing?" Lyndsey cried to the nurse. "He is in pain."

"No, no," said the nurse. "He's not really awake yet. He's not in any pain."

"Yes, he is." Lyndsey began to get hysterical. She did not know what to do. She started to shout. "Help him. Somebody help him. He is in pain."

They brought the hospital social worker to take Lyndsey out of the room. A little later, when she went back in, she heard Carter laughing with the nurses. He did not remember being in any pain. He was fine. Lyndsey got really angry.

"How could you do that to me?" she yelled at him. "How can you make me responsible for making sure you are not in pain?"

Carter admitted that it was probably impossible for Lyndsey to know whether or not he was in pain. "I'm sorry," he said, abashed, taking her hand. "I shouldn't have said that."

Lyndsey stormed out of the hospital. It was, she told me later, a very hard day.

*   *   *

At night, in the hospital where he was staying, Carter was having a dream. He was walking through the hallways of the hospital. Lakota spirits surrounded him. They were walking behind him and before him, dressed in their best ceremonial clothing. As all of them proceeded through the hallways of the hospital, there was an overwhelming feeling of love that came from the spirits into Carter. It was an ocean of love in which Carter dwelt, a powerful love that surged around him and inside of him. This was the love that the spirits had for Carter. Carter suddenly understood that the spirits had been walking with him his whole life. They had always been there. They had always loved him. He just hadn't known.

When he woke, Carter called Lyndsey to tell her the dream.

"I've wasted so much time," said Carter.

*   *   *

When Lyndsey told me Carter's dream, she started to cry. Poor Lyndsey, I thought. This was not what she signed up for when they got married. On the other hand, marriage was signing up for everything – the good and the bad, the sickness and the health. After all, what was love if it was not an act of courage?

"Lyndsey, you are so amazing," I said. "I am so grateful that you are there for him."

"He calls me his 'angel.' I hate that."

"Why? You know, you do seem fairly saint-like."

Lyndsey laughed. "Oh, please. I hate that. It is just not true. I can be a stone cold bitch."

"I don't know how you stand it."

Then she told me something that surprised me. "I'll tell you how I cope. I have a very powerful connection with God. Ever since I re-discovered God, I have strengthened that relationship with unending determination."

It was the G-word. She had religion, just like my friend Doreen. "I pray every day," Lyndsey continued. "Every day, I check in with God. I go to my meetings, too. And then there's my peer song circle." Each week, for several hours, four friends met with Lyndsey in the song room. There, they talked, prayed, and released their feelings from the body through vocalization – a spontaneous, wordless "river of song."

I remembered that once Carter and I went out on his boat on the lake when Lyndsey was having her peer song circle. He was uncomfortable. Their voices drifted out over the water as we pushed off from shore, tipping, our hands filled with rods and lures. The sun was spreading light above the trees, and a mist had risen from the water. "I can't stand listening to them," he said, rolling his eyes.

A voice lifted from a low tone to a fullness that seemed half song, half cry of anguish. Where were Carter's Spirits that day? We rowed out onto the lake, where the mist closed in around us. Heaven and earth were muffled, and we could hear nothing but the casting of our lines.

TWENTY-EIGHT: GOODBYE
December to May

*H*OW do you say goodbye? How many times do you say goodbye? It was the Winter Solstice, three days before Christmas. Four o'clock shadows lay across the hospital grounds. The air was crackling with cold, and it smelled like snow. Lyndsey got Carter from the hospital. He thought he was going home, but she took him straight to their town common. Lyndsey's sisters were there, her brother-in-law, her niece and nephews, and her mother. They were bundled up and standing on the green, waiting for Lyndsey and Carter. The children shouted for joy when he got out of the car. The children rode his scooter with him, and he tucked his niece, Lizzie, in front of him, guiding the scooter onto the green. It was their annual Winter Solstice caroling. Together, they lifted their voices in the songs of celebration.

Three days later, on Christmas day, Carter was back in the hospital. He was very ill, unable to keep any food down. A week later, he was home again.

All through January, February, and March, Carter went back and forth to the hospital. I began to prepare the children for the worst, but sometimes it sounded like Carter was getting better. It was confusing. Carter fought with the EMTs when the ambulance was called, and Lyndsey felt like she was going crazy. She was thinking about leaving; she wanted to run away.

By March, Carter was on regular dialysis. Fluid was drained from his abdomen once a week. His testicles began to swell again. Lyndsey called me, sobbing, from the hospital Intensive Care Unit. We think that this was it – the end. His blood pressure dropped to almost nothing.

But before we could rush off to Boston, he had rallied again.

That weekend, Lyndsey went on a retreat. The retreat theme was "Radical Honesty," and Lyndsey got honest.

"I think my husband is dying," she said, "and I can't take it any more. He gets better, he gets worse. He is in and out of the hospital every other day!" She had been crying so much, it felt like her eyes were going to fall out. The circle of others urged her to keep talking. "I've been thinking of leaving him," she admitted. "At the very least, I think I have to move downstairs into the guest room. I think I'm going crazy."

At the lunch break, three women from Lyndsey's group came and sat down next to her. They told her they were hospice nurses. "If you can get a doctor to admit there is nothing they can do to save Carter, you can get Carter set up with hospice care at home."

"But he doesn't have cancer. Isn't hospice is just for cancer and AIDS patients?"

"He doesn't need to have any particular disease; if it's terminal, you can get hospice."

"Well, obesity is definitely terminal," said Lyndsey, relief flooding her. Relief because, at that moment, she realized that she did not want to leave Carter. It was the stress. All the back and forth to the hospital; the long drives; the fear and the never knowing. At that moment, Lyndsey realized what a huge relief it would be if Carter could just stay home.

"At that very moment," she told me, "I loved him so much it hurt."

The next day Lyndsey drove to the hospital, filled with radical honesty and the hope of hospice at home.

"You know," she told Carter, "I've been feeling very angry. Angry and resentful, and scared it would go on and on. I'm so sorry."

"It's okay," said Carter, covering her hand with his. "I'd have felt the same thing if it had been the other way around. I'm sorry, too."

"But this hospice thing, this would be the answer to everything. All this back and forth to the hospital; it's just wearing me out."

They talked about how she would get the hospice service set up for him. "I will be there for you," she told him. "Even though our lives together didn't turn out the way I had hoped, God has given me one of the greatest gifts I could ever receive – the chance to be with someone all the way to the end of their life. I will not leave you to die alone. No matter how long it takes, I will be with you all the way. I love you."

"Thank you," said Carter, the tears sliding down his face. "I love you. I know –" his voice was broken, "you've been kind of – pulling away, and, I'm …" He breathed hard. "I'm so grateful for you …"

They couldn't go on. They talked about the hospice with great hope. Carter wanted to go home.

*   *   *

But no doctor would admit he could not help Carter. No doctor would admit Carter was terminal. How could you be terminal when there was no specific disease? How could you be dying of obesity? Day after day, Lyndsey tried to get the hospice care, but she could not. Again, she started getting very angry; she thought she would go mad. Carter went back and forth to the hospital. On May Day, Carter was home. Her family came for a Maypole Mayday celebration. Each person wrote a wish on a piece of paper and buried it in the new, spring soil under the Maypole. Lyndsey wrote; Carter wrote. They did not read each others' wishes; they both wished to be released from suffering. Two days later, Carter was back in the hospital again.

*   *   *

From the hospital, Carter called me. It was the only time he had ever called me first. "I realized I had all this prepaid cell phone time," he said, as if explanation were needed. "I wasn't using any of it."

Yes, I thought, I guess all our time is prepaid. Better use it while you can.

But he could not hold the phone to his ear. He was shaking and weak. He said his knees had buckled earlier in the day as he was standing at the sink to brush his teeth. It could be from the pain medications, he said. He was not sure what was happening, but he did not sound frightened. The phone fell from his hand and clattered to the bed. He picked it up. He said he had to call back. He had to call the nurse to put his headset on him. He hung up and called again five minutes later.

"Oh, that's better," he said, laughing. He sounded fine. I tried to imagine his giant hands so weak he could not hold a telephone to his head. I talked to him for a while. One by one, I called Harry, Byron, and Sean. We each spoke with him, telling him what we were up to. I watched the boys laughing. Uncle Carter was telling them something funny; I did not know what it was. Sean thanked him for the wonderful guitar that Carter had sent to him via Mom. It was a guitar that my father had given to Carter; now Carter was passing it along to Sean. We told him we loved him. We told him goodbye.

*   *   *

That day was sunny, gorgeous, and Lyndsey took the scooter and their dog, Tripper, to the hospital to see Carter. They all went outside to sit in the park in front of the hospital. No words were spoken; Carter just seemed to soak up the sunshine, the beauty and the warm, rustling presence of the trees.

That evening, as she left for home, Lyndsey looked back into his room. Carter seemed somehow smaller, lying back in his hospital bed, the bedside light in a pool on the night stand. He looked so tired, so lost and alone she thought her heart would break. But it had been a day of great beauty and peace. He was not afraid any more. He was letting go.

*   *   *

Carter died on a Saturday in May, a few days later.

I was annoyed as the phone rang before 6 a.m., waking me, even though it was time for me to get up to make the breakfast anyway. These thoughtless people, I thought, imagining that it was a B&B inquiry.

But it was Lyndsey, sobbing. "Oh, come right away," she cried. "I don't think he can last very long."

All the doctors had said he was stable, again; he was supposed to go home in two days. But he began to fail in the night. He was throwing up blood. Now, he was intubated. A respirator was breathing for him. He was already unconscious. "I am coming," I told Lyndsey. "I will be there as soon as I can. Call Caroline."

Lyndsey had tried to call Mom but she couldn't get through. After much consultation with Carter, Mom had gone to Texas to our cousin's wedding. We thought Carter was all right for the moment.

You always think that there is going to be more time.

Finally, I tracked Mom down in her hotel room. I'd woken her up, and she sounded disoriented. "I don't know if I can make it back," she said. "I thought he was going home this week. He kept telling me to go on to Texas."

"Ma," I said. "It's okay. He won't know the difference. He's already unconscious. You were there so much for him." I reminded her that we all had already said our good-byes. We'd been saying good-bye for months.

Still, it was terrible not to be there at the end. I didn't think I could make it in time. I told the boys I was pretty sure he was dying. Harry sobbed, and Byron was angry. I was distracted; I couldn't think. I helped Sean put out the B&B breakfast, then I left for Boston. I told Sean I had to go to the hospital alone. It was the final argument; it was the last goodbye, this most intimate encounter with death. This was between me and my brother.

But I was barely able to focus. I drove all the way to the next town before I realized I had forgotten my purse, and I had to go all the way back home for it. Caroline was on the phone when I got back, talking to Sean.

"He looks terrible," Caroline said as I got on the phone. She was in Carter's hospital room. "He is all blotchy, and his fingers are blue and his eyes are open, but he doesn't know we are here." She sounded shocked and frightened. She was there with Lyndsey and a friend of Lyndsey's and my niece, Emma. "I don't think he will last until you get here."

"Just keep him on the respirator," I begged. "Don't disconnect him. I want to be there before he dies."

They said they would not disconnect him, but he might die anyway. I was beginning to get a migraine and I had to eat. I drove through McDonalds, and then drove off in the wrong direction again. I had to turn around to go back. Finally, I got on the Interstate. After I'd been driving for an hour, the mobile phone rang. I pulled off the highway onto the shoulder to answer it. Cars blew their horns and whizzed by.

It was my sister. "He's gone," she said in a clogged voice. "He died at 11 o'clock."

Right around the time I was getting lost at McDonalds.

"Okay," I said, feeling nothing.

"He never woke up. I don't think he knew we were there."

"It was good you were there," I said. "I'm glad you were there."

"Yes," said my sister. "I'm glad we were here. What are you going to do?"

"I'm going to the hospital."

There was a pause.

"They've already taken his body to the morgue," said Caroline.

"I have to go to the hospital. I have to see for myself," I told her. "I want to see his body."

"The funeral home director may already have him by the time you get here."

"See if they can wait."

Caroline said she would try. She understood; for me, Carter was not gone. There was a scene in my mind, a frozen tableaux: Carter dying in a hospital bed, with Caroline and Lyndsey and Emma around him. It was burnt into my brain. And hovering around that bed was Carter. That was where I wanted to be. That was where I had to go.

As I drove on, the grief rose. Hot tears trickled down my face and turned into sobs. Sobs turn into louder sobs, and finally I pulled off the road again. I sobbed until I was not merely sobbing, I was yelling. I was actually screaming. Oh, my God, I was scaring myself! I sounded like a horror film. But it was the same when my father died. I was furious. I was enraged. I might have vomited on the floor, so sick was I with rage and grief. I grabbed the steering wheel and shook it, screaming and twisting, and gnashed my teeth, and kicked the floor, and cried and cried. Cars whizzed by, faces craned toward my car, but the curious did not stop.

Then, little by little, it died away. Screams died back into sobs. The sobs into tears. The grief into silence. The silence into peace. He had passed through me. I let him go.

I drove on and on. Lyndsey called me. Come home, she said. There is nothing at the hospital any more. Come home. She did not understand, either. I didn't argue with her, but kept driving for the hospital. I pulled into a gas station and called Sean, called my old friend Anne, and told them the news. Caroline called me. The funeral director called me. I no longer pulled over to take calls. The funeral director would meet me at the hospital. Caroline had arranged it for me. I drove on and on forever. Caroline had given me complicated directions – how to park near the front of the hospital, not in the rear lot. Yes, I had said, not listening. I already had my directions.

Then I was there at the hospital. Once inside the small entrance, the funeral director was easy to spot – a quiet man with a slightly bald head, looking for a stranger. He already knew I wanted to see Carter, and he went with an orderly to the morgue, and wheeled Carter's body out into a small, closed off hallway. I looked the other way until the two men had left through the swinging doors. Finally, I was alone with Carter.

Carter was on a gurney, in an unzipped body bag, and he looked very, very dead. I howled as soon as I saw him. Carter was definitely no longer here. This was a husk. He was in a black plastic body bag, unzipped to the chest, with his head surrounded by white plastic edges, so that he looked like a large black tulip, just blooming. His lips were pale and pulled down into an upside-down smile. His eyes were as shut as Caroline and Lyndsey could make them, a glisten lining the lashes. I felt the plastic; his arms and hands were crossed over his chest inside the body bag. His huge face was cold and waxen. There was blood on his nose. I leaned my head against his body, and I whispered goodbye.

The funeral director was very kind when I came out and thanked him.

"My brother held me up when I saw my father's body," I told the funeral director. "But now it is him."

I knew the funeral director didn't understand what I was talking about, but it didn't matter. He who had held me up was gone. This was just between me and death and the God that I did not understand.

After I left Carter's body, I found my way to the ICU where he had died only hours before. This was a tiny hospital, and it was not far from the morgue. It was very quiet in the ICU; there were no other customers that day. Three nurses sat chatting at the center desk, and beds with flimsy dividers curved around the edges of the circular room. As I entered the ICU, I began to cry again, and I held up a finger to the nurse, stepped back, turned around and tried to get control.

Control, however, was not forthcoming.

"I guess I'm not going to stop crying," I said to the nurses, turning back into the room. "So I guess I'll just come in."

I told them who I was and that I did not make it before Carter died. They showed me the bed where he had lain. It was near a window that overlooked a parking lot. Carter's blood pressure began to drop at 4 a.m., they said. They gave him medication to bring his pressure back up, but it did not work. Three times, they tried to save him. His organs failed, and his blood became toxic. He became groggy; he slipped into a coma. Carter asked the nurses to stay with him, so that he would not be alone. If only he had been at home with hospice care, I thought bitterly. One of the nurses had held his hand.

I cried, and the doctor hugged me. The doctor and his family were from one of those Muslim, middle-eastern countries, and I was a lapsed Christian from New York City. But such things did not matter when it came to love. Who were these men on the news that told us we were enemies? Who were these terrorists who thought they understood God? The doctor hugged me, and told me it was all right that I did not make it before my brother died, and I cried into his arms. I thought that perhaps there, at that moment, perhaps there I understood God.

Back again in the rear parking lot, outside by the car, it was quiet. The late afternoon sun was hot. There were no other drivers. I was not in the hospital visitors' parking lot after all. Unwittingly, I had broken the rules once again; I had parked where only doctors should be.

Do you mind? I am so sorry; I am sure you will forgive me.

I laid my notebook on the ground, found a pen, and called my sister. I didn't know where I was. As I sat on the warm tarmac, she gave me directions, told me how to get back home.

TWENTY-NINE: PICTURE THIS
May

*M*OM was angry when she arrived at Carter and Lyndsey's house, a day later. "I'm not going to cry any more," she had said sternly. "I cried all day yesterday, and I am finished crying." She had hugged me and pushed me away.

We were sitting on the nubbly carpet in the Song Room, where Lyndsey was going to hold the memorial service the next day. Lyndsey had asked Mom to choose photographs from boxes and albums, photographs of Carter to stick onto a big board for the wake. Some were very old – photographs Mom took of Carter as a child. Some were from the Peace Corps. Some were more recent. "I can't do this," Mom said angrily with a sniff. "What does it matter! What does it matter!"

"I'll do it, Mom," I said. "It's okay. You don't need to do this. I like to look at these pictures."

There was one of Carter from high school graduation; I was surprised to see he was thinner and very handsome. There were pictures of Carter fishing, pictures of Carter in the mountains, a recent picture of Carter at the May Day celebration, sitting on his scooter gazing down, the cherry blossoms thick above his head. Mom took the pictures from me and arranged them on the board.

"You don't need to do this, Ma."

"Well, how are we going to stick these on?" She ignored me. "Not this one," she said, discarding a picture. "This one." She chose a better snapshot.

We were preparing for a "new age" kind of memorial to be held after a brief wake. It was what Carter and Lyndsey wanted, but it was not very Episcopalian. Not what Mom would have done for her son at home in Connecticut.

"None of my friends in Connecticut knew him," Mom said angrily. She did not want to do another service at home. "What does it matter?"

Sean, the boys, and I went to the funeral home first, and to my surprise, it did not frighten me to see Carter. I was glad to see him. Carter lay in an open casket. He was not very made-up; he looked natural, even beautiful, dressed in the soft, white deerskin Native American costume he wore for his wedding, his fingers entwined in the medicine bag he held sacred. With my family around me, I dared to stroke his cool hand, touched a finger to his face. Were you allowed to touch the body? I didn't care. Harry knelt and prayed; Byron, the skeptic, did not.

Mom arrived with Caroline and my niece Emma. Caroline and Emma came in, but Mom did not. Caroline said Mom was "composing herself" in the car.

Caroline had never been to a wake before; she thought they were morbid. But when she sat next to me, she said, "Oh, I'm so glad."

"Glad?"

"He looks so much better. You can't imagine how terrible he looked at the hospital with all those tubes in him and his eyes open and staring like that."

I looked back at my brother. He didn't really look like he was sleeping; he looked like a lovely picture of himself, like a sculpture, or a reminder of who he was.

"Now I understand the wake," said my sister. "This is a good thing. I'm very glad this will be my last picture of him."

When Mom finally entered the room, she sat stiffly beside me without looking at Carter. She was dressed in white, the clothes she wore to the wedding in Texas. She did not glance in the direction of the body, but greeted people who came in murmuring condolences. Her eyes glistened. "Get a grip," she muttered to herself. I didn't recognize any of the visitors. They were here for Lyndsey. Harry sat crying, clinging to Sean; another of Carter's nephews, Dan, sat crying, too, clinging to his dad. Byron explored the funeral home, an antique Boston house, discovering history and touching things he shouldn't.

Slowly, Mom withdrew her camera from her capacious bag. "You know," she murmured to me, glancing at my face, "I'm going to take pictures."

"That's okay, Ma," I assured her, wondering if people usually took pictures of the dead body at a wake. I had been to only three wakes before, and nobody took pictures there. "Do whatever you want to do."

"I'm a photographer," she insisted. "That's what I do. I take pictures."

"That's good, Ma. You do what you want to do."

"I just want to let Lyndsey know," murmured Mom, afraid that she might shock somebody. "I'll wait till everybody leaves."

"Don't wait," said Caroline, sitting on the other side of her. "Look, nobody's in here now."

All of the visitors had gathered in the anteroom around the board with Carter's pictures and other memorabilia. "This is a good time," Caroline urged.

"Do you think …." Mom said weakly. "Don't you think I should wait?"

"No," Caroline directed. "Not till the end. Go ahead, do it now. This is a good time now."

Mom rose. A few people entered the room again, but she couldn't stop. The impetus of her need catapulted her forward. Mom approached Carter's body, the camera shielding her face.

"Uh, Lyndsey," I croaked. Lyndsey was embracing a friend, who spoke earnestly to her. "Uh, Mom's going to take some pictures, okay?"

"Huh?" said Lyndsey. She half turned.

The camera flashed.

Lyndsey watched.

Mom photographed Carter's body from the side, then from the foot of the coffin, then worked her way back up to his head. The children stared. I watched her small body, an older version of mine, tipping forward from its toes, the camera shielding her eyes, clicking. Flash, flash. She took her pictures; she lowered her camera to her chest and looked over the top of it at Carter, unblinking. And then her face trembled. Crumpled. The tears slid down her cheeks, dropped to the top of the camera.

"He looks ..." she said, sitting next to me again, blowing her nose with tissues.

"Beautiful," I said.

"Yes."

"I want to take a picture," said Byron.

"Me too. I want to take a picture," said Carter's other niece, Lizzie.

"Me, too!" The other children crowded in. "I want to take a picture." Mom surrendered her camera. All the children lined up to take pictures. Lyndsey laughed and cried at the same time. She circulated the room, embracing people, and the children stood on the brocade kneeling rack, taking turns with the camera.

Mom and Caroline and Emma and Sean and I talked about our last game of charades with Carter, and suddenly, we could laugh again.

"Oh, well," laughed Lyndsey, coming over to us wiping her eyes. She was a good sport. She sat next to me on the rickety wooden chairs. "I thought we would all line up here and sit on the chairs and greet people as they went by in a line." She laughed at her formal vision. "But I guess we're not doing that."

When we returned to the house, the food was all set out and the children were swimming in the lake, screeching and running around. It was wonderful to see and hear them being so alive. The day was gorgeous, the sun bright and warm.

Then the drumming began. Mom and I had just gotten our plates of food, and from below, in the song room, the drums were calling us to come.

"Uh-oh, Ma," I said. "They're starting the ceremony."

We went downstairs, balancing our plates of food. Inside the big song room, Lyndsey and her River of Song friends and the children (miraculously dry and dressed) and Lyndsey's relatives, Carter's best friend from the Peace Corps and some of Carter's former co-workers were packed in, sitting on chairs and on the floor, everywhere, banging drums with soft deerskin wrapped sticks. Small drums, larger drums, all handmade Native American drums. They were Carter's drums. Boom, boom, boom. The drums throbbed, pulsing and scary. I peeked into the room. Lyndsey's sister was picking her way between people, carrying incense that drifted into the corners. It smelled like marijuana.

Mom headed back for the door.

"I can't do this, CL," she said as I hurried after her, trying to keep the pasta primavera from sliding off my paper plate. "I'm sorry, I just can't do this."

"That's okay, Ma," I said. We went out into the sun and fresh air. Some people were still standing around, talking and eating. "You don't have to. Let's just sit here and eat our food." Somebody turned a couple of chairs around so we could face the lake.

Caroline and Emma were sitting nearby on the patio, just outside the song room, at the other end of the house. The large, sliding glass doors were open, and from the patio, they could see and hear the ceremony. "Come on over here," Caroline said, waving a hand. "Ma, sit over here."

We waved back and started eat. As the drumming throbbed louder and louder, Mom and I ate faster and faster. Then it stopped. We laid our plates on the grass.

Caroline was standing in front of us. "Mom," she said sternly, "you have to at least come over here where you can sit and see. It's rude!"

"All right, all right," said Mom, standing up.

I thought Caroline was being too bossy, but on the other hand, I didn't want to stay with Mom and miss the ceremony. I had my song to sing. "I'm going inside," I said. "Do you want to come in, Ma?"

"No, I'll sit over there with Caroline."

In the song room, the marijuana-smelling incense had dissipated and the drums had stopped. Sean was tucked away in the corner with Byron, and Harry was sitting near Carter's other nephew, Dan. Outside, Caroline was rearranging chairs. Mom sat just on the other side of where we'd had family therapy not so long ago. It was her turn to be backlit by the sun, the halo around her hair.

The center of the circular rug was filled with objects that people brought to represent Carter: photographs, sculptures, stones, feathers, letters, a fishing rod, a geode.

John, another nephew, read Carter and Lyndsey's invocation to the seven directions of the wind. Then each of us read, said, or sang something about Carter. When each person was finished, the group shouted, "Ho!" and banged the drums again. I got startled the first time it happened. "Oh," I said, jumping around.

"Mommy," muttered Harry. "It's *ho*, not *oh*!"

I was wedged between Harry's dinner plate and someone else's shoes. I saved the carpet from Harry's falling cup of soda and passed all the used paper plates along a row of hands to Sean, who was standing near the garbage can. The whole thing seemed pretty weird to me, but on the other hand, that was Carter.

But before I knew it, I was saying "Ho" with the rest, drumming my hand on my thigh. We sang and we talked about Carter. Mom sat outside the screen door, listening, nodding, the light glistening in her hair.

"I see Carter walking," said a man who claimed to be a medium. I didn't catch his name. ("The Large," Sean called him later.) The medium received messages from the Spirit World. He did not know Carter. He didn't know Lyndsey, either; I wasn't sure who even invited him. Somebody did invite him, though, with Lyndsey's permission, because earlier, at the funeral home, Lyndsey had thanked him for coming.

Evidently Carter was speaking from the dead to the medium. Sean, hackles rising, raked the medium with a glare. I was grateful that Sean didn't growl.

"And Carter has a star in his hand, here in the palm of his hand," said the medium, drawing a star in his palm. *Nice image*, I thought grudgingly.

As I was thinking about the medium's poetic potential, he said something else that I missed. He ended up touching his chest. "...From my heart," he said, gesturing toward Lyndsey, "to yours."

"Oh," Lyndsey cried out. "Oh! I can't believe it." She was very excited and her eyes were luminous. "Oh, I have to tell you all! This is so amazing. *I forgot this:* Carter said to me, he would send me a message if there was a spirit world. We agreed on our secret message. I forgot all about it until just now. We were watching television, and it was that commercial, you know, with the Pillsbury Dough Boy? And at the end of the commercial, the Pillsbury Dough Boy said, *'From my heart to yours.'* And he said to me, Carter said to me, *that would be his message!* If there really was a spirit world, he would get that message to me. *'From my heart to yours.'*" She gazed at the medium in awe.

Non-believer though I was, I have to admit that a chill or two tickled my spine. "He never even *knew* Carter," Lyndsey said of the medium. "I never met him before today. But that was Carter's message to me: *'From my heart to yours!'* Now I know! He really is here!" She rose with joy, looking up, tears flooding from her eyes.

"Ho," shouted the others, banging on the drums. The medium went on, talking about the "short one." "Carter says he is walking with the short one," said the medium. "Do any of you know who that would be?"

I was about to modestly rise and proclaim that it was probably me, when a friend of Lyndsey's, the one who took Lyndsey to the hospital and was there when Carter died, rose up and beamed at us.

"That is me," she says. "I am the 'short one.' " She was indeed short.

I was annoyed. Why was *she* the short one? Why not me? What, did Carter used to call her "Shorty" or something? I was, after all, just as short as she was. He didn't call me Shorty; Carter always called me "Ol' Four Toes," because one of my toes is deformed. Personally, I thought it was obvious that "the short one" Carter was walking with in the Spirit World must have been the Pillsbury Dough Boy, but this did not seem to be the general consensus, so I kept my mouth shut.

As I was debating in my head about the Pillsbury Dough Boy, I missed whatever it was the Short One said. It was just as she was finishing that I heard, "... and if you could sing the light Carter is walking in, it would sound like this."

Then she began singing one long note. She dropped to another note, took a breath, then rose to another long tone. It was haunting and beautiful, these notes from the heart without words. Nearby, I heard somebody mutter, "Tone jam." There was an excited rustle. Another voice joined in with the first, then another, and another, until everyone was singing long, chanting tones, harmonizing, weaving, some faster, some slower, taking breaths at different moments, the whole room dying low, then swelling loud again. I closed my eyes and lifted my face and the tones rose out of my middle where it hurt so much. I was not screaming now, and this was better than crying, this singing together. I could hear different parts of the room rising in different harmonies, dissonance and consonance at the same time.

It was a terrific release as we sang Carter's spirit up through the gates of heaven and perceived the light of Gabriel through our aural senses. The power of the River of Song shook the floor and the walls of the song room and vibrated right through me. We were rinsed with the Pythagorean muse – the worlds wheeled like ancient women, the vacant lots burned with poppies, and outside the song room, the May Pole fluttered with warm ribbons, leaving the cruelest month buried in the dust.

The song drew to a slow and natural close, and there was silence. Lyndsey stood and thanked everyone for coming. I woke, as if from sleep, refreshed and renewed. Carter and Lyndsey's rituals might be weird, but they worked for me.

But the day remained cruel to my mother. As everyone said goodbye and thanked each other, I went to Mom, out past the screen into the glaring sunlight, and hugged her. Light sparkled off the lake. She hugged me and pushed me away, smiling, gazing out at the lake. Behind us, the medium was still standing in the center of the song room, sobbing. He was becoming hysterical. Others were patting him, trying to calm him down.

"Jeez," muttered the overly perspicacious Byron, peeping back into the room, "why is he crying? He didn't even *know* Uncle Carter!"

Mom shook her head. "That man is a *nut*!" she said. She picked up her camera and stalked off to the kitchen.

Later on that night, as I struggled to stay awake, Sean revealed that he was awed by the ceremony.

"I never understood the importance of rituals before," he said to me when we were in bed. His face was all lit up with cosmic consciousness.

"Uh," I said, jerking my head up off the pillow and stretching my lids wide over my tired eyeballs. Why did men always get inspired to communicate at the most inopportune times?

"I thought having a wake was morbid. But now I realize I was afraid. I was always afraid I would say or do the wrong thing. But this was great. It was liberating. Nothing anybody could say or do was the wrong thing. And the singing together at the end, that was amazing. I never heard anything like it before."

The intensity of his feeling surprised me. Sean's musical tastes, while eclectic and broad, didn't lean in a New Age direction. But I knew what he meant: The experience was a way of expressing the grief and the joy, and of course, for men, emotions were dangerous. Emotions could threaten a man's self-image, his control, his pillar of strength.

That was where Carter had been a pioneer, a lonely frontiersman: He ventured again and again into that forbidden territory, trying to port his feelings out by whatever means he could discover or invent. He believed that without the willingness to go to forbidden places, man's strength was little more than a pillar of salt. I was glad my husband went with Carter on his last journey, this ceremony Lyndsey and Carter planned together before Carter died.

"I think *you* are amazing, Sean." I gave him a kiss, and he smiled and turned away, abashed, and stuck his nose into the latest *Scientific American*.

THIRTY: WINNING AND LOSING
June

$\mathcal{N}$OT long after we returned home, both Byron and Harry had simultaneous baseball games in adjacent diamonds on the same field. I ran from one fence to the other, cheering them on.

Between innings, I finally got a chance to talk to Byron's coach. "Carol, remember that day, that game when Charlie kept pitching balls and walking players?" I'd been burning to ask her this question. "Remember when he was crying, and you walked out there to the mound and talked to him? What did you say?"

"Oh, yeah," said Carol. She shrugged. "Nothing much, really. The usual. I just told him to relax, throw straight, you can do it." She grinned. "You know, like that."

Relax. Throw straight. You can do it.

On the baseball field, Byron's team was winning, but Harry's lost. The first two times at bat, Harry was terrific. He singled and stole all the way home. He sailed another one into the outfield. Then he flubbed it. He swung at pitches over his head and struck out twice. The team lost, narrowly. It was a good game.

"I can't deal with him," I told Sean. I was afraid I was going to get depressed. Harry was going to throw himself at my feet and tell me what a horrible week he'd had. First his uncle died and then he lost his baseball game, and his life was miserable and worthless and nothing made him happy. Oh, God, I couldn't stand it! I never knew you could spend all this time and money and energy on yourself to become mentally healthy, only to suffer all of the same awful feelings through your children all over again. "I have to go to book club," I said. "You tell him to stop being so miserable. Take them out for ice cream."

But I didn't escape in time. Harry was hiding in the van – my getaway car – crying his eyes out. Privately, I admitted to myself that it did suck that their team came in last place last year and wasn't doing much better this year. But what could you do?

"That's it," said Harry. "I stink!"

Sean and I got into the van and launched simultaneous frontal and broadside assaults.

"What are you talking about, *'I stink!'* " Sean said indignantly. "You do not stink. Look how much better you are than last year. You hit better. Look how hard you can hit this year. You catch better."

"Yeah," I added. "Look at all those catches you made in the outfield in the second inning. Those grounders. You used to miss those last year."

"You have to learn from your mistakes," said Sean. "If you go around saying, *'I stink,'* you can't learn anything!"

"The competition is not with the others, Harry," I adjured him. "It seems like you are competing with others, but that's really not the point. The competition is with *yourself.* What am *I*? Who am *I*? Can *I* improve? Can *I* do better than I did before?"

"It's not *fair*," Harry said angrily through his tears. "This was supposed to be my year! This was supposed to be the year we won! And now," he buried his face in his hands, his thin shoulders shaking with anguish over the consequences of losing, "we will *never* get our free ice cream."

I frowned at him. " Harry, your team played a great game. Focus on the positive, not the negative. Look how well you did at first. You got a single and stole all the way home! You were the only one to score in that inning!"

"Yeah, then I struck out twice!" he added bitterly.

"Hey!" Now I was shaking my finger. Now I was giving orders. Now I was Mrs. General Mommy Watson ordering my son to arms. "You stop feeling sorry for yourself. You focus on the positive. And you learn from your mistakes."

"Yeah, you made a mistake," Sean said. "Who doesn't make mistakes? Your mistakes are a gift, Harry. That's how we learn. That's how we get better."

"You were the only one to score in the first inning, Harry," I added. "Remember that. *The only one!*"

Then, miracle of miracles, a tiny smile fluttered at the corners of his downturned lips. A thimbleful of pride glanced from his eyes. My heart soared. If only he knew how desperately we cared. If only he knew how scared we were! If only he knew how completely we loved him.

"Hey, hey," I said, tickling. "I see a smile. I see a little smile there trying to get out."

He giggled. He was okay after that. Not going to commit suicide today. No, no, not going to become a drunk today. Not gorging ourselves today. Not going crazy today. Did we help him? Did we lay a brick down in the foundation of self-esteem? I just didn't know. We do our best, like most parents. We hope so.

Later, at book club, I sang my brother's song to my friends. Instead of talking about our book, we discussed addiction in the family. Everybody had a story. "I did my share," said Norma. "I'm no saint. But after a while, I realized this wasn't doing me any good and I quit. But my brother just couldn't stop."   Norma had lost her brother to suicide a year ago; he was a cocaine addict. "That's my question," she said. "Why can some people pull back from addiction, and others can't?"

That was my question, too. Why did I make it, and my brother Carter didn't?   The other women decided that the difference between the person who became a hopeless addict and the person who could save himself was a matter of self-esteem. You had to value yourself enough to get the help you needed, my friends said. In the end, you had to have enough self-esteem to let go of your addictions.

But I was not sure. Self-esteem was important, but it sounded too simple to me. What about humility? What about honesty? Just what was this "self-esteem" thing, anyway? In school these days, they told all the children they were wonderful no matter what they did, and that was supposed to give them self-esteem. But what kind of a self were you learning to esteem? A fearful self? A deceptive self? A lazy self?

What if self-esteem didn't give you the courage and honesty you needed to get straight; what if, to the contrary, courage and honesty gave you self-esteem?

It all went back to the theory of dog-mind. You had to discover your true place in the pack. You had to be willing to fight. You had to roll around on the floor and see who came up on top. You had to sniff and growl and mark your territory. You had to tuck in your tail and lie down when you were whipped. You had to be willing to lead when you won. It was all about balance, about having all four feet on the ground. You had to dig up the courage to lose, and you had to eat crow before you could win. You had to embrace the dead as well as the living and roll around in the smelly ephemeral stuff of the earth to become a happy dog among dogs.

Our kids were not the best athletes, nor were they the smartest students, nor were they the most handsome at the party. But then, neither were most of the other kids, and I tried to think, sometimes: What could we all tell our children that was true; how could we encourage them without making things up? How could I give them a foundation to fight the good fight? How could I help my kids break the cycle, to move into a happier, healthier life than my brother lived? What might any parent say that was true for every single child?

You are unique. You are special. You are amazing.

For what else do we tell them and show them, again and again, but that we love them? This ineffable beauty of the individual spirit made flesh, of which I am a part and I observe from a distance at the same time.

And was it not what Gandhi said to the Hindu: that he should adopt the orphan child of a Muslim, and raise the boy in his own faith, so that the man might come to see the unity in the body of his family that Gandhi himself longed for in the body of India? And was it not Martin Luther King, who learned at Gandhi's feet, who said that we should judge not by the color of the skin but by the nature of the heart? And what fear drives men on to such destruction that these messages of love must be ripped out of the world with bullets and buried in political careers? What fear drives us on the lee rocks of the wind, where our unity cannot endure the pounding of our hearts?

My brother was afraid, and he did not have the courage to face himself. Did my parents do their best with Carter? Did they make him feel less than loved? Could I possibly blame my aged mother, bearing up under grief, for being too distant and demanding in her prime? Could I blame my tortured father, dancing himself to death, for not being there at all? Or should I blame the twist of fate and sheer genetics? Why did Caroline and I survive, and Carter did not?

All I know is what I believe, and I believe that the decision to be honest with yourself is a choice. I believe that we all start out prisoners to our natures, and it is only by dint of hard effort that, little by little, we become free. Freedom is a choice, a personal decision. True, some people get more help than others along the way, but in the end, whether or not you hoist yourself up by your own collar or let yourself sink into the muck – it is really all up to nobody else but yourself.

I had hoped to end this account with me sitting next to my brother, with Carter reading this book while I sat next to him, waiting for him to say, *Yes, this is okay, you can publish this.* He would have liked this book, I was sure. He would have given it his approval. He would have laughed and he would have cried. He would have hugged me and told me he loved me.

So instead, I will end this saga with something small, but something not at all inconsequential. I will go to the secretary in the office at Byron's school, and in some quiet moment between children and teachers and telephones, I will look her in the eye, and I will say, *I feel that I have done something to offend you.* And I believe that she will be honest with me. I will grit my teeth and take it when she tells me some incourteous remark or bombastic mistake I have made. And I will think about it, and try to see it from her point of view, and I will try to learn from it and become a bigger person.

And if she says, with some surprise, *Oh, no, not at all, I am not angry with you, that isn't it, that's not it at all,* then I will think about T.S. Eliot's ragged claws, and that fear, and that honesty, and we will keep on talking. And I believe we will at last speak our separate truths, and from that moment forward, we will be more and better connected, that secretary and I.

At such a moment, the past will thin to a transparency, and in the gloom, in the half-lit living room, my father will sit smoking, listening to Mahler, the smoke curling round his wrist and lifting like the tongue of some ancient complaint. At such a moment, I will tell him what I wanted to tell my brother, what I want my sons to understand: *You are unique, special, and amazing.* And if the faith that you are loved can give you the courage to look to your true self, then may all the laurels of the world weigh for eternity upon some other brow.

Because I believe that most people, in truth, yearn for nothing more than love and connection, but only are afraid, and that at heart, most people in this world want to be good. We only have to find the place where we can meet.

THIRTY-ONE: ABOUT OBESITY

Recovery and the Family

L OOKING back on what happened has helped me realize that our "intervention," or family-therapy meeting, did work. My brother might have gotten better. After the family meeting, he did embrace a new attitude. I think Carter felt inspired by our meeting, and he came to believe he could get better. He found a diet that worked for him, and he found a new goal: to lose enough weight to enjoy a wilderness rafting trip once again.

I say, my brother *might* have gotten better, but there was one thing stopping him: It was too late. Therein lies the tragedy of our family. We waited too long; we took action far, far too late.

By the time Carter was ready to recover from compulsive overeating, his heart and other organs were too damaged. Finally, when Carter's spirit began to recover, his body was too frail to follow.

I am convinced that if we had seriously intervened earlier, we might have saved Carter's life. I will always regret the fact that after our family reunion in St. Louis, years before Carter's heart attack, when I realized Carter probably had angina, I did nothing about it.

While it is true that nobody can make an addict stop, it is equally true that an addict cannot stop (or stay stopped) alone. I believe that loving confrontation by a group of people the addict cares for and trusts can make the kind of difference that nagging, threatening, cajoling, and reasoning cannot. And although intervention is not always successful, it may plant the seeds of a later recovery.

Fortunately, a food-addicit does not have to recover alone. There are organizations that create a community of "abstinent" eating such as Overeaters Anonymous and Weight Watchers and various Internet communities. I believe that involvement in one of these organizations, together with a supportive family environment, can help a compulsive overeater regain a healthier relationship with food.

Perhaps obesity is so intractable, so difficult to beat because it is an addiction that many doctors still treat like a character defect or a bad habit. If we were to treat obesity like an addiction, an obsession of the mind and spirit as well as an illness of the body, perhaps we would see more success without surgery.

Finally, I would like to say that my opinions are based solely upon my own experiences with alcoholism, compulsive eating, and obesity. Take what seems useful and leave the rest. It is my hope that our family's story will inspire others to get healthy before it is too late. And if you do find success in overcoming this terrible disease, please take a moment to think of the brother I couldn't save, and his favorite Lakota prayer: *"Mitakuye Oyas'in*: Health and help to all my relations."

The Epidemic

*E*VEN though many medical professionals study and treat obesity in a subspecialty called "bariatrics," this killer disease is still little understood. In his address to a National Institute of Health (NIH) congressional subcommittee, Dr. Michael Jensen, a Mayo clinic doctor and then-president of the North American Association for the Study of Obesity (NAASO) testified that federal funding for obesity research is far too small to fight this growing epidemic – only one percent of NIH's total research budget (NAASO, March 6, 2002).

And obesity is an epidemic. In the year 2000, obesity was responsible for as many as 300,000 premature deaths and cost the nation some $117 billion. According to a 2002 Harris Poll, 80 percent of Americans over age 25 are overweight. That's an increase of 58 percent since 1983. One-third of all adult Americans are obese – again, the numbers have doubled since 1983 (Harry, H., 2002). Obesity is the number two preventable killer of Americans, right behind smoking. And as more and more of us give up smoking, obesity is rapidly becoming number one.

What is obesity, exactly? First of all, it is different from being overweight. Being overweight is unhealthy, but obesity is the point at which a person's weight causes serious and measurable health problems. There are two ways obesity is gauged. For some time, the measure of obesity has been a weight 20 percent or more than "ideal body weight." ("Ideal body weight" is the weight that is right for optimum health, calculated according to height.)

More recently, obesity is measured as "Body Mass Index," or BMI. BMI, measured with the metric system, is your weight (in kilograms) divided by your height (in meters) squared. You can go to one of many websites that calculates BMI for you, such as http://www.cdc.gov/ nccdphp/dnpa/bmi/calc-bmi.htm. A BMI of 25 or more is considered overweight. A BMI of 30 or more is considered obese.

Obesity increases the risk for about 30 serious medical conditions, including cancer, heart disease, Type II diabetes (which can lead to other serious illnesses and organ failures, such as kidney failure, blindness, and limb amputation), high blood pressure, stroke, gallbladder diseases, asthma, osteoarthritis, depression, sleep apnea, and complications in pregnancy. Health problems linked to this killer raise an individual's health care costs by 36 percent and medication costs by 77 percent, exacting a higher financial toll on health than either smoking or drinking (Sturm, R., 2002). The life-span of a man who is morbidly obese at age 25 is about 22 percent less than that of a normal-weight man (Fontaine et al., 2003).

The story is even scarier when you see what is happening to our children. Between the 1960s and 1980, the number of children who were overweight and obese remained about the same. However, between 1980 and 1999, the prevalence of overweight and obesity in children ages 6 – 11 doubled, and for adolescents age 12 – 19, overweight and obesity *tripled* (NAASO, March 6, 2002; CDC, 2002).

Doctors are seeing more and more Type II ("Adult Onset") diabetes in children – a type of diabetes linked to obesity that, until recently, was seen almost only in adults. For a growing child, the overweight body is sometimes too great a burden for the bones and cartilage. Obesity can cause serious orthopedic problems for children, like bowed, overgrown leg-bones and problems in the hip joint growth plate (AOA

Fact Sheets).

Studies show that parents underestimate the health risk of overweight in their children. They don't understand, either, how difficult it is to get their children to change and behave in ways that might prevent obesity. And no longer does this battle belong only to America. Obesity is becoming a worldwide epidemic. Obesity is a growing problem for children and adults in countries such as Egypt, Mexico, and even some Sub-Saharan nations. Over half the world's newly diagnosed cases of diabetes come from India and China (McLellan, F., 2002).

Causes

*W*HAT is causing this epidemic? One study finds that obesity is spreading to developing nations where there are rapid changes in technology, urbanization, transportation, and processed foods (Friedrich, M., 2002). Research indicates that it's not the fast-food franchises that are globalizing obesity, but rather the pervasiveness of low-cost sugar and edible oils, together with shifts in technology and transportation that decrease physical activity.

"Slow metabolism" and "hormones" have been claimed as a cause for obesity, but most evidence shows otherwise. For example, a study of Pima Native Americans indicated that only about 12 percent of obesity could be attributed to metabolic rate, but 40 percent could be related to eating and lack of physical activity (Ravussin & Bogardus, 2000). In 1995, researchers discovered that leptin, a protein [hormone] produced by human body fat, crosses the blood-brain barrier and informs the brain that there is plenty of fat in reserve. In other words, leptin tells the body to stop eating (Leptin, 1995). But as an anti-obesity medication, Leptin worked only for the 5 percent of obese people who could not produce this hormone naturally. The other 95 percent of obese people, who had plenty of leptin already, kept eating (Lane, L, 1999).

NAASO, citing a study by Tardoff (2002), speculates that the mere abundance of sugary drinks may be contributing to America's obesity epidemic, noting that teens may consume up to 1,000 calories a day in sugary soft drinks (NAASO, Feb 26 2002).

While genetics may contribute to an obesity predisposition, a CDC survey study demonstrates the fact that genetics is not the only cause. The study shows that while there was a significant change in the prevalence of obesity between 1991 and 1999, the U.S. gene pool did not significantly change during that time. These results demonstrate that "genes related to obesity are not responsible for the obesity epidemic in America" (Mokdad, AH et al., 2000).

But what about the fact that obesity, like alcoholism, tends to run in families? Obese people are 2 to 8 times more likely to have obesity in the family than non-obese people, and the more seriously obese the individual, the more likely it is that there is obesity in the family (Perusse, 2000). Such findings lead many researchers to look for a genetic link.

Genetics & Addiction

*T*HE medical establishment believes that genetics plays a role in obesity, but no one understands exactly what that role is. In rare cases, variation in certain genes clearly leads to obesity. Obesity is a "feature" of more than 30 genetic disorders (WEBmd, 2002). But for most obese people, the genetics of the problem is less defined. Does a certain genetic configuration lead to one person feeling less full and more hungry, while another feels more satisfied with less food? Does a certain genetic configuration lead one person to *enjoy* food more than another, to get more pleasure out of food?

The pleasure centers of the brain involve the neurotransmitter, dopamine. There are certain parts of the brain that work specifically to "receive" dopamine, and when they do, there is a "reward" sensation in the body. In fact, in a study of dopamine and cocaine, Volkow found that increased brain dopamine significantly correlates with an increased perceived "high." In other words, the more the dopamine, the greater the high (Volkow, ND, 1999).

Not only is brain dopamine increased by "psychostimulants" such as alcohol and cocaine, but it is also increased by "natural" rewards such as food and sex. Hernandez & Hoebel (1988) hypothesized that the dopamine reward-system stimulated by eating could be a factor in food-addiction. In fact, just being *near* food can trigger the dopamine system, which may help explain why people overeat (Volkow, ND, 2002).

By the 1990s, a dopamine receptor, the Taq1 minor (A1) allele of the DRD2 gene, was recognized as an important genetic factor contributing to alcoholism. Might this genetic factor also contribute to compulsive overeating and obesity?

A review of the scientific literature suggests that there is some kind of genetic similarity between alcoholism and obesity. On a personal note, I believe that my brother's obesity was directly related to, or a manifestation of, the alcoholism in our family and that genetics played a role in his food-addiction. His illness puts me in mind of what I call the "kaboom" factor. The phrase comes from an audio tape my father bought years ago, after he got sober in Alcoholics Anonymous, a tape called *A New Pair of Glasses* by Chuck C. In this tape, Chuck C. talks about his recovery from alcoholism. He was on the wagon but he still wrote advertising for liquor, and he suggested to his client a slogan something like this: Drink so-and-so liquor. It goes *kaboom!*

The client looked puzzled. "Kaboom? What are you talking about, kaboom?"

"You know," said Chuck C., who was also perplexed. "The way, when you drink it, you feel this big *kaboom!*"

The client shrugged. He didn't know what Chuck C. was talking about. He had never gotten a *kaboom* from alcohol.

That's when Chuck C. realized for the first time that other people, regular non-alcoholic drinkers, didn't necessarily get a *kaboom* from booze. And the *kaboom* he got from alcohol might have something to do with his alcoholism.

The scientific hypothesis goes like this: Because of some kind of genetic deficiency in the brain's dopamine system, substance-abusers may seek to stimulate the reward section of the brain by other means. In other words, non-addicts with normal dopamine reception apparently get the kaboom-factor on a regular basis and from all sorts of natural things. However, they may experience it at a somewhat lower intensity: an ongoing burble of pleasure, perhaps, instead of an occasional kaboom. Addicts with abnormal dopamine reception don't get the dopamine "reward" on a regular basis. Since the addict isn't getting much of a reward sensation, he goes for the gusto. Pour it on! Pour it on more! Eat! Eat! The dopamine levels soar. *Kaboom!*

Prevention

*W*HATEVER the role of genetics, obesity is a growing epidemic because modern culture promotes all the things that lead to food-addiction and obesity. Thus, the cure for the obesity epidemic is for us to change modern culture. Cultural change is not impossible; it just takes some time, money, and effort. I can think of several state or federal initiatives that might help: Ban sugar from school foods and drinks and give kids fresh fruit for dessert and snack. Have gym five days a week. Ask schools to screen all children and adolescents for obesity and enroll families in anti-obesity programs. Start an anti-obesity campaign as vigorous as the anti-smoking campaign. Make soda cans carry large warning labels about the dangers of diabetes: WARNING: THE SURGEON GENERAL HAS DETERMINED THAT CONSUMING LARGE QUANTITIES OF HIGH-SUGAR BEVERAGES CAN CAUSE LIFE-THREATENING ILLNESS

Federal initiatives should also include a centralized agency to combat obesity. There is a tremendous fragmentation of the medical and health establishment when dealing with this health issue. Federal initiatives are spread out over the Centers for Disease Control, the Office of the Surgeon General, the Office of Disease Prevention and Health Promotion, the National Institutes of Health, the Food and Drug Administration, the US Department of Agriculture, the Federal Trade Commission, and the Department of Health and Human Services. Citing this fragmentary, sometimes redundant approach, the American Dietetic Association has called for the creation of a well-funded, single institute to study the causes of obesity and factors leading to successful treatment (Dausch, J, 2002).

The growing trend in America and in the worldwide community seems to indicate that the problem is something more than a "lack of empowerment," as the federal government often seems to imply. Federal initiatives must do more than "empower" us with education and pep talks. How about spending some *money* on this issue? Good exercise must fit into the rhythm and flow of a modern life, and the federal, state, and local governments can help make that happen. Create sidewalks for kids to walk a couple of miles to school instead of bussing them. Mandate sidewalks for rural roads. Build a federal network of bike paths across the nation's rural regions. Provide tax-incentives for companies that provide their employees with a gym or special time for workouts. Build federally funded weight-loss community centers with ongoing weight-loss programs and exercise facilities for *families*, not just adults.

Treatment

*I*N the past few decades, treatment of obesity (excluding surgery) has become more successful than it used to be. After losing weight, however, the problem becomes keeping it off. In the 1950s, it was thought that 95 percent of people treated for obesity gained the weight back. These days, according to Dr. Jensen, half the patients enrolled in long-term programs commonly manage to achieve and maintain weight loss that has significant health benefits. Several research studies have shown that increasing physical activity is absolutely essential to maintain a weight-loss that results from dieting. Researchers can even specify the amount of physical activity necessary to prevent gaining the weight back (Jensen, M., 2002).

More recently, bariatric surgery, in particular Roux-en-Y gastric bypass surgery, and to a somewhat lesser degree, gastric banding, has been found to be a successful treatment for morbid obesity (BMI over 40, or BMI over 35 with other illnesses). Studies show that both short- and long-term, surgically treated patients lose a substantial amount of weight and have a better quality of life. One study showed an average 25 percent weight-loss maintained after ten years for patients who underwent gastric bypass (Sjöström, L. et al, 2004). In about 75 percent of gastric bypass patients, Type II diabetes disappeared completely, often within days after surgery (Buchwald, H. et al., 2004). On the other hand, surgery can result in death or painful complications; at the very least, it means a tremendous, sometimes difficult life adjustment. Of significance, several studies show a "steep learning curve" for bariatric surgeons (Courcoulas, A. et al., 2003; Giusti, S. et al., 2003; Maggard, M. et al., 2005; Weiner, R. et al., 2003; Zingmond, L. et al., 2005).

Surgeons who performed fewer operations (less than 20) had a higher patient mortality rate than those who had performed more operations (greater than 250). There were fewer patient complications in hospitals with higher volume (more than 200) than in hospitals with lower volume (less than 100) (Courcoulas, A. et al., 2003; Zingmond, L. et al., 2005). Finally, the types and techniques of bariatric surgery have been refined and improved over the years, lessening the mortality rate as well as the number of post-operative complications.

Toward a Healthier Future

*W*HILE surgery has become an increasingly popular way to deal with morbid obesity, the obesity "epidemic" cannot be stopped by surgery alone. We need to deal with the behaviors, attitudes, and foods that are causing the problem.

My personal opinion is that obesity is an intransigent illness because it is not merely a physical problem, but is – at least in some cases – like alcoholism, an addiction. To beat addiction, most people must experience a profound shift in attitude. And what treatment will provide this deep change, this complete willingness, this foundation upon which to build a new and healthier life – especially when everything around you encourages you to eat too much and exercise too little?

The first step toward more effective treatment is, I think, awareness – awareness that obesity should be treated as an addiction. Second, effective treatment must offer an abstinent community environment, such as the OA or Weight Watchers community, in which the food-addict can live, eat, and socialize without having temptation set under his nose. Third, it has been demonstrated that the parents of overweight children and adolescents must be involved for a successful treatment; the reverse is probably true for adults. Effective treatment should be a family affair, not an individual diet, and diet programs should be structured to incorporate the extended family or even the workplace, if possible.

Fourth, a daily lifestyle change that incorporates more physical activity is necessary, and as a nation, we should spend the money on making that possible.

BIBLIOGRAPHY

(AOA) American Obesity Association. Fact Sheets. http://www.obesity.org, accessed 2002.

Blachar, A et al.: Gastrointestinal Complications of Laparoscopic Roux-en-Y Gastric Bypass Surgery: Clinical and Imaging Findings. Radiology 223:625-632, 2002.

Buchwald, H et al.: Bariatric Surgery: A Systematic Review and Meta-Analysis. JAMA 292:1724-1737, 2004.

Buchwald, H and Williams, SE: Bariatric surgery worldwide. Obes Surg.14(9):1157-64, Oct. 2004.

Center for Disease Control: Prevalence of overweight among children and adolescents: United States, 1999. National Center for Health Statistics 2002 April. http://www.cdc.gov/nchs, accessed 2002.

Christou, NV et al.: Surgery decreases long-term mortality, morbidity, and health care use in morbidly obese patients. Ann. Surg. 240(3):416-23, discussion 423-4, Sep. 2004.

Clegg, AJ et al.: The clinical effectiveness and cost-effectiveness of surgery for people with morbid obesity: a systematic review and economic evaluation. Health Technology Assessment 6:12, 2002.

Courcoulas, A et al.: The relationship of surgeon and hospital volume to outcome after gastric bypass surgery in Pennsylvania: a 3-year summary. Surgery 134(4):613-21, discussion 621-3, Oct. 2003

Dausch, JG: The obesity epidemic: What's being done? J Am Dietic Assn 102(5): 638-9, May 2002.

Dymek, M et al.: The quality of life after gastric bypass surgery: a cross-sectional study. Obesity Research 10:1135-1142 , 2002.

Executive Order on Agency-wide Activities to Promote Personal Fitness. White House web site (http://www.whitehouse.gov/news/releases/2002/o6/20020620-4.html), accessed 2002.

Fontaine, KR, et al.: Years of life lost due to obesity. JAMA 289: 187-193, 2003.

Forwood P, et al.: The genetics of addiction: alcohol-dependence and D3 dopamine receptor gene. Pathol. Biol. (Paris):49(9):710-717, Nov. 2001.

Friedrich, MJ: Epidemic of obesity expands its spread to developing countries. JAMA 287(11):1382-6, March 20, 2002.

Gustavsson, S & Westling, A: Laparoscopic adjustable gastric banding: complications and side effects responsible for the poor long-term outcome. Semin. Laparosc. Surg. 9(2):115-24, Jun 2002.

Harry, H: The Obesity Epidemic Is Getting Even Worse. The Harris Poll ® #11, March 6, 2002 @ http://www.harrisinteractive.com, accessed 2002.

Harvey, SC, et al: The GABA(A) receptor alpha1 subtype in the ventral pallidum regulates alcohol-seeking behaviors. J. Neurosci. 22(9):3765-75, May 1, 2002.

Hedenbro, JL and Frederiksen, SG: Fully stapled gastric bypass with isolated pouch and terminal anastomosis: 1-3 year results. Obes. Surg..12(4):546-50, Aug 2002.

246

Hell, E et al.: Evaluation of health status and quality of life after bariatric surgery: comparison of standard Roux-en-Y gastric bypass, vertical banded gastroplasty and laparoscopic adjustable silicone gastric banding. Obes. Surg. 10(3):214-9, Jun 2000.

Hernandez, & Hoebel, BG: Food reward and cocaine increase extracellular dopamine in the nucleus accumbens as measured by microdialysis. Life Sci. 42(18):1705-12, 1988.

Jensen, M: NAASO address to National Institute of Health congressional subcommittee: May 2, 2002 http://www.naaso.org, accessed 2002.

Kothari, SN et al.: Lap-band failures: conversion to gastric bypass and their preliminary outcomes. Surgery 131(6):625-9, Jun 2002.

Lane, L: What happened to leptin? WebMD, 1999 August 30: http:/www.cnn.com/HEALTH/diet.fitness/9908/30/obesity.gene.also/index.html, accessed 2002.

Leptin helps body regulate fat, links to diet (press release): Rockefeller University, 1995 October 31: http://www.rockefeller.edu/pubinfo/leptinlevel.nr.html, accessed 2002.

McLellan, F: Obesity rising to alarming levels around the world. The Lancet 359(9315), April 20, 2002.

Melis, M, et al: Long-lasting potentiation of GABA ergic synapses in dopamine neurons after a single in vivo ethanol exposure. J. Neurosci. 22(6):2074-82, Mar 15, 2002.

Mokdad, AH, et al.: The continuing epidemic of obesity in the United States. JAMA 284(13):1650-1, Oct 4, 2000.

Noble, EP: The DRD2 gene in psychiatric and neurological disorders and its phenotypes. Pharmacogenomins 1(3):309-33, Aug 2000.

Noble, EP: Addiction and its reward process through polymorphisms of the D2 dopamine receptor gene: a review. Eur. Psychiatry 15 (2):79-89, Mar 2000.

(NAASO) North American Association for the Study of Obesity: NAASO responds to recent Harris poll on obesity, March 6, 2002 http://www.naaso.org/newsflash/harrispoll.htm, accessed 2003.

(NAASO) North American Association for the Study of Obesity: Sugar Drinks Rapidly Converted into body fat, study shows. February 26, 2002 http://www.naaso.org/newsflash/2_26_02b.htm, accessed 2003.

Perusse, L: [Genetics of human obesity: results from genetic epidemiology studies] (French) Ann. Endocrinnol. (Paris) 61 Suppl 6:24-30, Dec 2000.

Ravussin, E & Bogardus, C: Energy balance and weight regulation: genetics versus environment. Br. J. Nutr. 83 Suppl 1:S17-20, Mar 2000.

Ritter, MM: [Obesity is not a character weakness. Leptin and twin research show: fat control is genetically regulated] (German) MMW Fortschr. Med. 141(49-50):28-30, Dec 9, 1999.

Sjöström, L et al.: Lifestyle, Diabetes, and Cardiovascular Risk Factors 10 Years after Bariatric Surgery. N. Engl. J. Med. 351(26):2683-93, Dec 23, 2004.

Sturm, R: The effects of obesity, smoking, and drinking on medical problems and costs. Health Affairs 21:245-253, 2002.

Suter M: Laparoscopic Roux-en-Y gastric bypass: initial 2-year experience. Surg. Endosc. 17(4):603-9, Apr, 2003.

Tardoff, MG: Obesity by choice: the powerful influence of nutrient availability on nutrient intake. Am. J. Physiol. Regul. Integr. Comp. Physiol. 282(5):R15369, May 2002.

Thome J., et al.: Genome polymorphism and alcoholism. Pharmacogenomics 1(1):63-71, Feb 2000.

Volkow, ND, et al.: Reinforcing effects of psychostimulants in humans are associated with increases in brain dopamine and occupancy of D(2) receptors. J. Pharmacol. Exp. Ther. 291(1):409-15, Oct 1999.

Volkow, ND, et al: "Nonhedonic" food motivation in humans involves dopamine in the dorsal striatum and methylphenidate amplifies this effect. Synapse 44(3):175-80, Jun 2002.

Weiner, R, et al.: Outcome after laparoscopic adjustable gastric banding - 8 years experience. Obes. Surg.. 13(6):965, Dec. 2003.

WebMD: Genetics of Obesity. DNA Science article. July, 2000: http://www.cssvc.health.webmd.compuserve.com/content/article/2731.431, accessed 2002.

Zingmond, L et al.: Characterizing the performance and outcomes of obesity surgery in California. Am. Surg. 69(10):823-8, Oct 2003.

Special thanks to David Little Elk, who interpreted Carter's Lakota prayer, *Mitakuye Oyas'in,* which means "all of my relations." David says that the full spiritual meaning of *Mitakuye Oyas'in* is, "Everything is connected to each other in the universe within myself, just as I am connected to the universe outside of me. Thus, what I do, feel, say, and think affects that which is around me. And by Natural Law, it returns to me four times as strong as when I first sent it out. So when I communicate in a good way, it returns to me stronger. When I communicate in an unhealthy way, I only hurt myself more than others." David Little Elk's web site is http://www.malakota.com

Special thanks to Sean Nixon and his SUNY Ulster design class for work on the cover of this book.

RESOURCES

Addiction Intervention Resources at http://www.addictionintervention.com

Al-Anon Family Group at http://www.al-anon.org

American Obesity Association. 1250 24th Street, NW, Suite 300, Washington, DC 20037 (800) 986-2373 or (202) 776-7711. http://www.obesity.org

BMI (Body Mass Index) calculator at http://www.cdc.gov/nccdphp/dnpa/bmi/calc-bmi.htm

Internet search using the key words "binge eating disorder" yields many useful results.

National Health Information Center, P.O. Box 1133, Washington DC 20013-1133 (800) 336-4797 or (301) 565-4167 http://www.health.gov/NHIC

National Institute of Diabetes & Digestive & Kidney Diseases (National Institute of Health), Health Information, Weight Loss and Control http://www.niddk.nih.gov/health/nutrit/nutrit.htm

North American Association for the Study of Obesity. NAASO Executive Office, 8630 Fenton St. Suite 918, Silver Spring, MD 20910 (310) 563-6526   http://www.naaso.org

Overeaters Anonymous at http://www.overeatersanonymous.org

Residential weight loss center at http://www.structurehouse.com

River of Song Workshops with Lyndsey Watson at http://www.riverofsong.com

Weight Watchers at http://www.weightwatchers.com